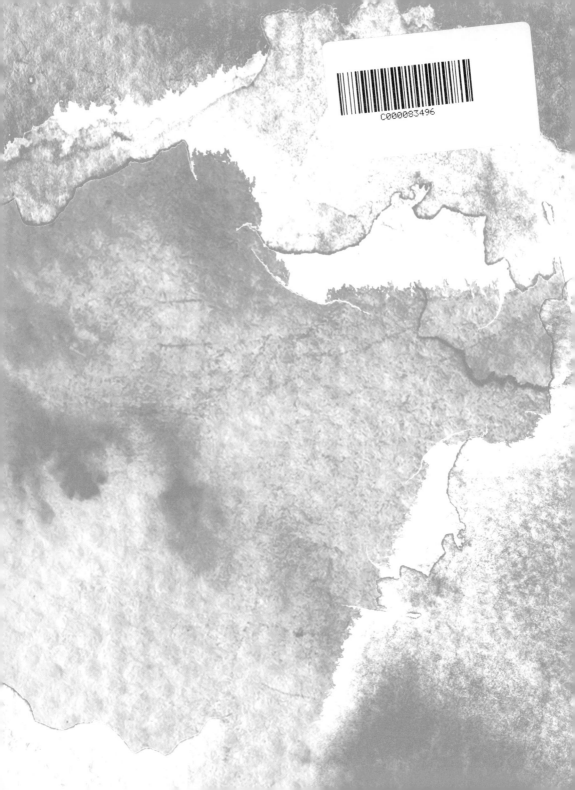

The Making of YOU

The Making of
YOU

a guide to finding your identity and bossing motherhood

Binky Felstead

PIATKUS

First published in Great Britain in 2023 by Piatkus
1 3 5 7 9 10 8 6 4 2

ISBN 978-0-349-43379-0

Book design: Hart Studio
Photography: author's own

Printed in Italy by Printer Trento Srl
Papers used by Piatkus are from well-managed forests and other responsible sources.

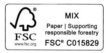

Piatkus
An imprint of
Little, Brown Book Group
Carmelite House
50 Victoria Embankment
London EC4Y 0DZ

An Hachette UK Company

www.hachette.co.uk
www.littlebrown.co.uk

For Max, India and
Wolfie – without whom
this book could never
have been written.

Contents

Introduction

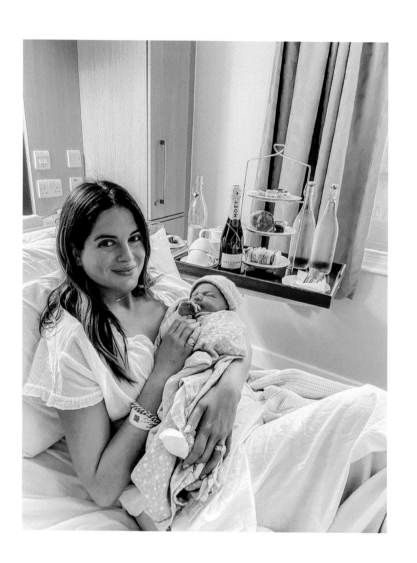

From the moment you become a mother, your life will never be easy, predictable or smoothly go the way you expect it to again. Will you still be effortlessly glamorous and spontaneous like you could be in your pre-parent days? Probably not. Will you be tired and confused? On many days, sadly, yes. Will this new version of you feel a love deeper than you ever imagined, and will your days be touched with wonder and beauty? Oh God, yes – but it *will* all be a bit messy and exhausting as you shape your family into the healthy, happy unit you are determined to build. That's reality. And that's what I'm here to help with.

Let me share a very real example of this straight from the delivery room, seconds after I'd given birth to my second child, my son Wolfie. He'd arrived pink and squealing, gorgeous, after an 11-hour labour, and we were in that exhausted glow of unrequited love that washes over you when you meet your child for the first time. The midwife asked my husband Max if he'd like to cut the umbilical cord. He didn't want to really, I could tell, but he felt pressured to be at least some part of the physical process after watching me squeeze and strain and sweat a human being out of my vagina for the last few hours, so he reluctantly took the scissors . . . and just as he moved round to the end of the bed to make the snip, my placenta flew out and up, through the air, before landing on the floor next to his feet with a thwack, splattering everyone within 2 metres of its landing spot with blood. It was like something from a horror movie – it was humongous! Disgusting! Our happy smiles twisting into disturbed grimaces!

And Max still has the blood stains on his trainers. The brand-new, bright white trainers he'd just bought. I don't think he'll ever wash the blood off. I don't think he'll ever wear them again, either, because that would be stinking gross. But as he says, those trainers are a very, very gruesome reminder of a very, very lovely day. And that's parenthood and family life right there in one anecdote. It's mucky and magical, funny and fleeting, difficult and delicious. Working hard to make my family work brings all those things to me every single day. Mostly, though, it brings gratitude.

Why gratitude? Because struggling with the lows of mothering – and relishing the highs – has also been the making of *me*. It has changed me, given me clear purpose, and made me feel wholesome in a way I didn't know would ever be possible after years of being bullied as a child, living through my parents' difficult divorce as a teenager and being on reality TV in my twenties. Being a mother has grounded me and made me the happiest I have ever been in my life.

I'll share a secret with you. Before India came along, I didn't really know what I was doing. I was going out and having fun, being a typical twentysomething, drinking until I fell over then waking up with anxiety attacks. I had no idea what I could do or become. I didn't have any qualifications, so knew I was never going to be a brain surgeon or become Prime Minister. I never went to university because my mum, affectionately known as Mummy Felstead, had said, quite rightly, that paying for me to

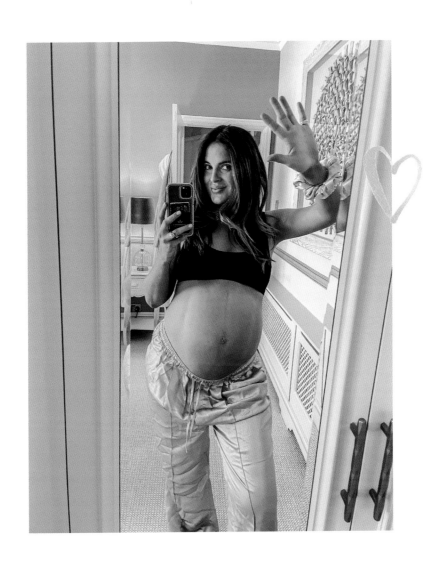

study for a degree would be like tearing up £10 notes and throwing them into a fire. After school, I did odd jobs and internships, showing up for interviews in Ugg boots – which I didn't know was unacceptable – then got my first job as a receptionist at Candy & Candy, which was great fun, then at a hedge fund, where I answered the phones and slept off my hangovers on the sofa while the bosses were out to lunch . . . I fell into *Made in Chelsea* – which was tremendously lucky of me, and fun – but everyone knows celebrity is fickle and oftentimes shallow, and too frequently leads to even more insecurities and self-doubt than before the fame, money and adoration gets handed to you on a silver platter . . . And that's where I was when I became a mother to India, aged twenty-six, in the public eye, and the first of my friends to get pregnant and have a baby.

After the shock, the solicited and unsolicited lessons started flooding in. Motherhood taught me who I am, what is important to me, and it's given me the drive to be as successful as I can so that I make my kids proud. I want to make my own money so India knows how it's done. I want to collaborate on big ideas so I'm a role model for Wolfie. I've never been more inspired; I've never been more fulfilled – and too often in the day-to-day grind, exhaustion and swapping of war stories about the hardships of motherhood, we forget the lessons and blessings. I'd love *The Making of You* to be a reminder that every shitty moment as a mum has a glorious silver lining if we simply know where to look.

Even though I was (I am!) a young mum, I felt ready. I was the one who played with dollies, and who was naturally good with babies, since being a baby herself. I can't remember a time I didn't dream of being a mother. I wanted, and still want, the country house crammed with kids, supper warming in the Aga, ducks and chickens running around outside while I teach the children how to make daisy chains in the shade. I suppose I want to replicate the family life of my early childhood. I can still vividly remember the safety and joy I felt when I was really small, having a bath in our old country home with the window open to the garden, feeling the sun streaming through on to my skin, listening to the birds tweeting their merry song, and smelling a bonfire from across the fields. It gave me a warm rush then and it still does now – the happy family home of my childhood is still somewhere I take myself to when I'm feeling low or uncertain, and I'd love to give that to my children. That desire gives me direction.

And of course, the legend that is Mummy Felstead informs how I mother, too. Growing up, my mum had an open-door policy where her friends were always welcome for a glass of champagne while their offspring – my friends – were running wild and stealing drinks. Mummy was an amazing hostess, always looking so pretty and serving delicious feasts. We had the best parties. She was definitely a cool mum, and I really enjoyed that. She still is to be fair! As fans of *Made in Chelsea* will remember, she was always entertaining my friends, in on the gossip.

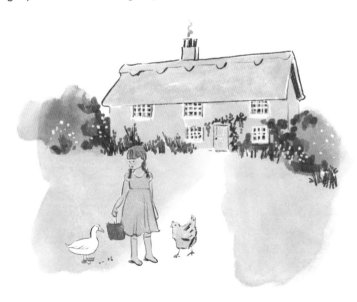

Things did take a downhill turn when my dad lost his job, and my parents got divorced when I was a pre-teen. Suddenly I'd find my once gregarious, excitable mum crying in the bathroom, and our privileged life was constrained. It felt like life had suddenly got much tougher but it wasn't that dramatic. We never wanted for anything, but life felt very different to what I'd been accustomed to for the first ten years of my life. Two things kept me going. Firstly, I was happy to still be able to visit the pony I'd ridden since I was little, as mucking out in the mornings lent consistency to my daily routine, and it got me out of the house, so I didn't have to hear the arguments. Secondly, Mummy and I grew incredibly close – we still are today – and I learned a lot about motherhood during that time, about how to enjoy it and create those safe spaces that turn into fuzzy lifelong memories . . . and how to survive the tougher moments.

Through any trauma, I remember having carefree, sunny days with my mum – picnics on the beach, rock pooling, paddling, and that is what I want to give my children, not the five-star resort-style holiday that money and guilt buy. My favourite moments with my children are our morning walks to a nearby pond to feed the swans, long lunches in pub gardens, dancing to 'We Don't Talk About Bruno' in the kitchen while I make roast chicken. I don't want my kids to be spoiled.

At heart, I'm just a mother who doesn't understand her children sometimes; a girl next door who sometimes finds herself dressed up on red carpets but would rather be watching movies on the sofa snuggled up with her family; a woman who frequently makes mistakes like everyone else, and gets back up because she has to – and that's what I want to share with you in this book about my experiences of life and motherhood. Max is the same. He isn't a posh boy, he's a proper grafter, and he grafts just as hard to make our family work as I do, despite setbacks, hurdles and pitfalls.

Maybe that's what I *most* want to get across in the pages of *The Making of You*. There is no easy route to being a perfect mother or raising perfect children. In fact, there is no such thing as perfection. *But* you can try hard to make it work in a way that allows your family to be as happy and healthy as possible. Try your best, put in some effort and don't beat yourself up. Ask for help. I have! Not only from my family and friends but from people who I will gladly admit know more about parenting than me. I'm blessed to have access to the UK's most brilliant pregnancy, motherhood and medical experts on Bloss, the app I set up with another amazing mama, Steph Desmond, and I am so excited that many of them are sharing their educated insights, bright ideas and pearls of wisdom with you here in this book. In each chapter, along with my personal anecdotes, angles and anxieties, these extraordinary leaders in their field will share easily digestible information to help you navigate not only how you parent but how you look after yourself, too.

At the back of the book, you'll find a notes section for you to journal about your own experiences and jot down any pointers that might help you. I find writing lists and affirmations helps to encourage me to make good decisions and keep me on track.

I'd argue – as would this wonderful tribe of experts – that looking after your own mental and physical health is probably the most important thing you can do as a mother. I've known so many women over the years, close friends – boss ladies who are so strong and powerful in other areas of their life – who beat themselves up over minor issues, struggle mentally because they are afraid to ask questions, allow external judgement to depress them, or second guess their instincts as a mother to the point of derailment. Of course, there is a spectrum of struggling mentally and emotionally post-partum and through parenthood and knowing when to seek help is crucial. In the back of the book I have listed some useful resources in the UK.

Please also speak to your family, midwife, GP, etc. Help is available, even if it sometimes doesn't feel like it.

As an example, just the debate about whether you breastfeed or not is so loaded and harmful during those first few days – even hours! – of motherhood, when women are tired and vulnerable. Yes, breast is best but, for God's sake, give yourself a break and do what *you* want or need to do! It's perhaps not fashionable to think about yourself – but that's where I've always been grateful for the straight-talking common sense that I've got from Mummy. Early on with India I was a mess one night because she wouldn't sleep, so I couldn't sleep, because she wasn't full enough and I felt I had to keep trying with my boob, and in an old-fashioned, brilliant way, Mummy said, 'Give her a bottle, it'll be fine.' And it was, and we both slept. She did the same when in those first few weeks I felt I couldn't let India leave my sight for a second. Mummy insisted I could and should take 10 minutes to go and have a hot shower, wash my hair and, of course, we all survived.

Do-gooders and naysayers may encourage you to second guess every decision you make as you parent your child. I felt that pressure, I do understand! But think about it: you've made some good decisions in your life up until this point, right? And no one loves your child more than you. Trust your gut rather than following the crowd. Ask people you trust for their opinion, but don't listen to everyone's because you'll go mad.

Don't just look for guidance on social media. If you're feeling a bit shit and down on yourself, heading to social media will make you feel bad. Strangers displaying their curated best bits is a sure way to make you feel even worse about your own life. Even people you know can make you feel lesser – there's a mum I know who is always posting videos of her looking glamorous and her child looking neat as they bake cakes, which makes me second guess myself – especially when I know she's not like that in real life. Block, mute, delete and look away, especially in moments of mothering self-doubt.

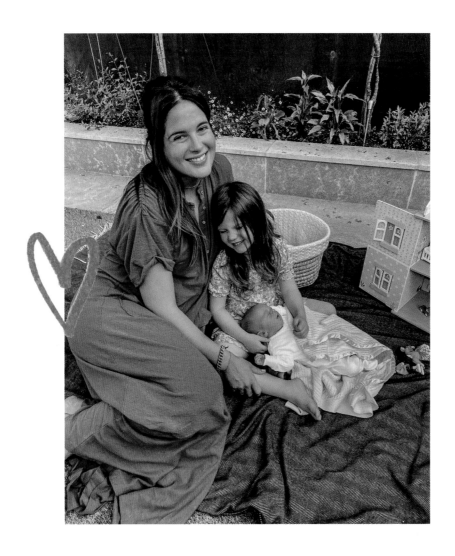

I remember going on *This Morning* when India was a brand-new baby and getting so much abuse on Twitter about how I was holding her, it was really hurtful and unjustified. Any judgement can hit hard. This book is here to remind you to keep focused on yourself and your own family; your version of good might look different to everyone else's and that's okay.

Try to enjoy motherhood! Enjoy the gang you've created. Be the boss of the family business. I never felt worthy or like I belonged until I became a mother. I was a loser at school, bullied and lacking in confidence. I was shocked I was chosen for *Made in Chelsea* over dozens of other girls who were prettier, slimmer, more fashionable; confused that the producers saw something in me that I didn't see in myself. India made me grow up and realise for the first time in my life that I didn't have to give two shits about anyone else. It was me and her against the world. She was born on 12 June 2017, and I turned twenty-seven just two days later. I had no idea at that point that I needed her as much as she needed me. But she truly changed my life for the better, despite the sudden changes to my freedom, my social life, my identity, and that her father and I split up just over a year later. For a year, India and I were a strong twosome, doing everything together, forging a bond we'll have for ever, although it's adapted to our new life with our two boys, Max and Wolfie.

Whatever your current circumstances, things are going to be okay. That's the hope I want *The Making of You* to bring you. If you're trapped in a relationship that isn't working, know you can leave – you're not alone any more, you have your child. If you're raising your child alone, there's magic in the closeness you'll find together. If you're single and unhappy about it, read my story. It took another single mum writing to me on Instagram, warning me about hiding myself away – just when I'd met Max – that pushed me to take a chance and go on a date with him . . . and the rest is history. This book will provide snapshots of positivity wherever you are on your motherhood journey.

And the main thing you'll get from me, and the experts whose advice will be shared throughout the chapters, and that I hope you'll find in yourself as the book prompts you to consider your own life as a mother, is gratitude – an appreciation for the things you get to experience as a parent. A business conversation might have gone badly, but when I take India for a walk in the sunshine and she gasps at the beauty of the trees, it reminds me to stop and appreciate small, simple pleasures too. You get to watch your child watch the world, and that's a privilege that has made me happier than any money, or fame, or fancy gift. And if this sounds a bit twee or rose-tinted, do know that I fully expect to mess up my kids in some way. Just ask any therapist. We try our best, but we'll still mess them up somehow – and I know, because I've had lots of therapists myself, that the mother always takes the lion's share of any blame – but my children make me want to learn, to improve, to make them proud, and they make me excited for the future. And I hope this book will help you celebrate the life you've made for your family – whatever shape, size or situation it is currently in! You can make it work.

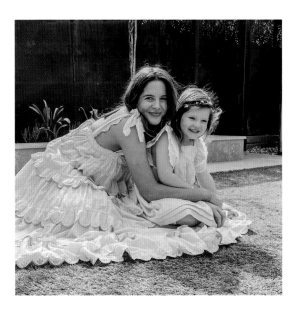

CHAPTER ONE

The Last Trimester

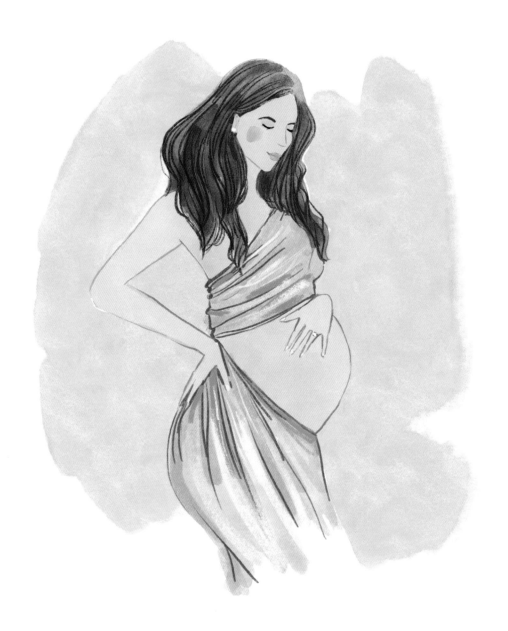

My final stages of pregnancy with my two children couldn't have been more different. Being pregnant with India came with a lot of chaos and mental exhaustion. Mixed in with the excitement about meeting my little girl was fear and nerves, like most first-time pregnant women I'm sure, but especially because it very much wasn't planned. I was the UK ambassador for Reebok at the time I got pregnant, so I was really training hard, and thought that was why I wasn't getting any periods. It was my mum that suspected something when I'd gone out for a big fry-up breakfast and couldn't touch it – even though I normally eat like a horse – and made me take a test. Off we went to the pharmacy, and luckily bought a couple, because I peed on the wrong end of the first one. The second test stick showed I was pregnant. A scan at nine weeks confirmed the news. The *Made in Chelsea* producers wanted to get the news out before the paparazzi broke the story, so rushed to shoot a new scene of me showing scan photos to Rosie Fortescue, Stephanie Pratt and Louise Thompson, but the news broke before the cameras had finished rolling.

That night, India's dad and I went to The Shard for dinner to celebrate our news – we were the first reality television couple to have a baby, so it felt exciting for so many reasons. It felt like the whole of England was celebrating this with us. But then things got a bit more real. He and I were filming a two-part spin-off show to *Made in Chelsea* called *Born in Chelsea*, so I was being watched and listened to, prepared for public consumption the whole time, and my flat was being renovated so there was crap piled on top of crap on every floor while the builders kept getting further and further behind. I had no mental or physical space in which to relax or to nest, and that is all I wanted to do: prepare for my baby. I was overwhelmed and pissed off, obviously hormonal and just wanting to get everything in place, which was impossible. I felt trapped and confused for a lot of that last trimester, so the birth was actually an endpoint I was nervously looking forward to.

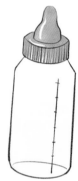

Mummy Felstead gave me the best bloody advice ever when it came to delivering India. Knowing I'm terrified of pain, and like to be organised, she told me that if I was ever going to spend money on anything, it should be on delivering my baby in the best way possible (for me!), with as predictable a birth as we could manage and an epidural, picking the date and the doctor. I didn't want India popping out on my birthday, so I chose two days before, and got induced – and she ventured out with the help of a doctor, Tom Setchell, whose father Marcus had delivered me, my brother and my sister decades earlier. He was also the Queen's gynaecologist and delayed his retirement to safely deliver Prince George, which is quite cool. The birth bit was fine . . . it was the aftermath I didn't love, my forced entry into a negative mummy club with unsolicited advice about how I'd never brush my teeth or have a shower again.

I brought India home from the hospital on my birthday, to a flat full of carpenters banging and clattering away, and I just burst into tears. I told them to leave and Mummy calmed me down with a cup of tea. Friends came over and did all those annoying post-renovation tasks that needed doing – like putting cutlery back in the drawers – and I had help to get India's nursery ready. Everyone says you should always add on three months to what the builders originally say because they're all assholes, so my advice is don't move or decorate in your last trimester. It's a major disruptor.

I couldn't openly lose my shit though, because the birth was in the press and I knew everyone was watching me. It was intense, but a cool time. My house was so full of flowers it looked like someone had died, and there were enough cakes being sent to set up a bakery stall on the pavement outside. But after those first few weeks of excitement when everyone wants to meet the baby, it all quietens down, and it's just you – who has had zero sleep – and a tiny little human, navigating this new life together. The flowers are dead and need to be chucked away; the cakes have all been eaten and you feel bloated, you're realising your boyfriend is still going to the gym or work every day, while you're at home in a tracksuit and you don't love it . . . and then the hormones really get crazy, your boobs are sore and leaky, and you're not getting the support from your partner that you need. It can be bloody hard.

My second last trimester

My pregnancy with Wolfie was a different ballgame because I was settled and content with Max, and already knew what to expect. I had a lovely time eating beige carbs and not caring because I knew I was loved – and I wasn't being watched so intensely by the media. Max is a very cool, dry guy – he's very Virgo, super-organised – which made me feel secure and looked after. He did lots of practical things in those final few weeks before my due date, like planning the route to the hospital and how to use the baby car seat, he even went and found the nearest parking spaces so I wouldn't have to hobble far to the entrance of the hospital. One thing he couldn't prepare for though was how much he was going to fall in love with this new little human, and that was fun to observe. He knew he was having a son, because instead of reading the gender result for our scan, I forwarded the email straight to a friend who filled a balloon with blue confetti which we popped in front of our family in the kitchen. It was fun to listen to him talk about the plans he had for the future, the moments from his boyhood he'd recreate for his boy.

I got induced again with Wolfie, as I had been for India, so we made our way to the hospital calmly – although Max's parking plan didn't work out, and we ended up having to leave the car in a road scattered with syringes, and prostitutes and pimps running around barefoot. I remember thinking our car would have been turned into a drug den or knocking shop on our return, but at that moment I didn't care. We just grabbed my hospital bag and rushed off. With India, everything happened within a couple of hours and I thought that would happen again. It didn't. This labour lasted for ever, and I was so tired and drugged up I couldn't even open my eyes and certainly didn't want to move, until – finally, after what felt like an age – this amazing midwife called Mona forced me to get up, get in position, and told me to push when I got the push sensation.

I was so out there, but I remember Max holding my hand throughout, telling me stupid jokes to try and make me laugh and take my mind off the fact I was pushing a giant thing through my vagina. And then Wolfie was here – and I saw tears in Max's eyes – and I remember that feeling of having a baby placed in my arms for the first time and doing that instinctive check for ten fingers and ten toes . . . and that overwhelming instant love I'd felt once before with India swept over me – but this time, without any fear or worry about what was to come next. Then of course my placenta flew out

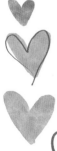

28

and ruined Max's trainers, and he went down to the lobby for the pizza he'd ordered just before Wolfie had come out, because I was starving and hadn't eaten all day.

I was exhausted after the long birth. When the nurses offered to take Wolfie to the nursery so I could sleep that first night, at first I felt too guilty to accept but Mummy Felstead came to the rescue again. 'He won't remember, don't be so ridiculous,' so I let him go and got the rest I needed. It wasn't just the labour that had worn me out but the few months before labour, when I'd had pregnancy insomnia and a constant need to wee throughout the night. 'You're not going to sleep properly the rest of your life,' she continued. 'Grab help when you can.' I'm glad I did because when we went home from the hospital, I didn't get an undisturbed night's sleep for a long while. And you know what they say: happy mum, happy baby. I am a much better mummy when I'm rested. We probably all are. Try to avoid falling into those guilt traps, often forged from those comments other people make about us or our parenting. If your child is safe and loved, that's good. You don't need to be with them and on it 24/7. You do still need to be you – and feel human – you know!

———

One thing he couldn't prepare for though was how much he was going to fall in love with this new little human.

———

WHY YOUR WELLBEING

MATTERS MOST AS A MOTHER

AIMEE STRONGMAN, YOGA TEACHER FOR BIRTH
AND ANTENATAL EDUCATION

According to the Royal College of Obstetricians and Gynaecologists, 'As many as one in five women develop a mental health problem during pregnancy or in the first year after the birth of their baby. The pain this causes women and their families, the negative impact on their health and wellbeing, and the economic costs to individuals, the NHS and the nation are considerable.'

Mothers are fundamental to a child surviving and thriving and their wellbeing truly is at the heart of society. The impact of motherhood is life-changing, brain shifting and heart bursting. It is a rite of passage that we just don't value enough in my opinion. Wellbeing in motherhood matters because this transformation affects every part of life. There are seismic shifts in the brain, in the body and, I would argue, the heart too. Birth is big and mothers need all the support they can get to make this transition from maiden to mother. If we don't take care of our mental health by seeking support or activities to keep ourselves balanced it is not just us that is affected but our children and partners too. We are the most important people to our children, and it is necessary that we protect ourselves in order to protect them.

Motherhood can be really isolating. Hours spent feeding a new being, new feelings, new routine, no sleep – it's hard. I began my business in April 2020 when all services to pregnant women and new mothers were stopped. I saw the need for the support, having a young baby myself, and felt offering my time and virtual space to help build and create our own support village was really essential. Since then, I have provided yoga classes, antenatal courses – both in person and online – new mother wellness walks (collaborating with my local NHS GP surgeries) and offer mother and baby circles as a way to gather as a collective in the early stages of motherhood to come together, share, listen and support without judgement or expectation.

My top tips for during pregnancy include writing a list of self-care activities you can do in 5 minutes (brush my teeth and add some mascara), 20 minutes (shower and make-up), 45 minutes (warm cup of tea, magazine and phone scroll) and 1 hour (walk around the block). Then when the baby arrives, you'll know things you can do to help take care of you!

—

As many as one in five women develop a mental health problem during pregnancy or in the first year after the birth of their baby.

—

IGNORING THE OPINIONS OF OTHERS

One downside from my delivery day with Wolfie was the negative comments I was getting online. The company I was helping to run at the time wanted me to post progress videos on the website, so our experts could offer advice in real time, so I put up on Instagram a video of me having contractions . . . and the wolves came out. *'You're not showing a real birthing story because you're obviously doing gas and air!' 'You're cheating! You're on pain relief!'* Yes, but I'm still bloody well pushing a baby out, I thought, and not dealing with my pain doesn't make me more of a mother, or in less of a traumatic situation! These judgemental mothers who try to pull down other mothers really piss me off . . . Please don't pay attention to them. They have too much time on their hands, or they're jealous – whatever it is, ignore them. Just listen to experts, friends and family who you trust. I've had to get strong in that respect, since becoming a mother, otherwise I'd go mad. Because it never stops – from whether you breastfeed or don't (I mixed with formula from day one), to if you send them to playschool or not, to what you let them wear when they're teenagers. Just make sure that what you are doing is right for you and your child. And never be that spiteful woman who throws shade at other parents. Keep it to yourself, unless your advice is specifically requested. Most people are kind, and I got much more positive feedback on social media than negative, but you always remember the nasty comments and it can really break your mood.

PREPARING OLDER SIBLINGS

After the birth – and my flying placenta incident in the delivery room – the four of us settled at home in a blissful bubble. I think the ease India felt came from the way we'd prepped her during the last trimester. We'd had a miscarriage at nine weeks before we got pregnant with Wolfie, so I was apprehensive about when to share our news with India, but as my tummy got bigger and bigger, there was no hiding a baby was on the way. To involve her, we'd gone to the shop and she'd purchased her future brother a Sophie la girafe toy, which she was excited to hand over, but I'm not sure she actually 100 per cent understood what was going on until she met Wolfie.

There's two pieces of good advice about introducing a child to their new sibling that work: make sure you're not holding the baby when they first meet, give the other child a hug immediately, so they don't feel stung by the replacement, and prepare a present from the new brother or sister in advance. All kids love presents! I filmed India meeting Wolfie for the first time, in the garden. We laid out a picnic blanket on the grass and placed him in a little basket on it in the shade, with a gift he'd bought for her – a doll's house – and waited for her to get back from her father's. To her credit, the love and excitement was instant, and she just kept asking if we could really keep him. It's a big deal for an older sibling to understand how their family will change, and what they can expect.

Another tip I have for that first meeting, one I was grateful to receive, was to remind visitors coming to see the baby to be excited to see the older child too – ask questions, be affectionate, bring a treat or a gift – and even think about keeping a little trinket box to present the siblings with something to make them feel special if the visitors are wholly focused on the new arrival. I really feel we handled Wolfie's arrival well because India is lovely with him, and she thinks of him as 'her baby'.

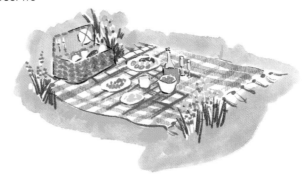

HELPING YOUR CHILD
BECOME THE OLDER SIBLING

MICHELLE TANGEMAN, LICENSED THERAPIST AND CREATOR OF THRIVING TODDLER

Introducing a new baby to the family is a big change for your toddler. Here are some ways to support your older children as you prepare to bring another child home.

BEFORE BABY: Select age-appropriate books to read together. There are many great books, but my daughter and I especially enjoy *Hello in There: A Big Sister's Book of Waiting*. My then two-year-old loved seeing the belly and baby grow as we turned each page. If you have the time and energy, creating a personalised story is a great primer for the changes about to happen. There are several reasons why I recommend this: it's personalised with images and text specific to your family's needs and it's something tangible they can hold on to and request to read with you as needed.

AFTER BABY ARRIVES: It's hard to know how each of your children will respond to the new family member. Scheduling special one-on-one time with your toddler may help minimise challenging behaviours that come up when attention is directed away from them. Be specific with your toddler about how you want them to interact with the baby. When Covid came as my youngest turned three weeks old we didn't know anything about the virus so we were very specific on how our toddler could interact with the baby. We told him that she could rub his feet, touch his belly gently, and kiss him on the head. This also works to your advantage when you have a really active toddler who is handsy. Always notice and point out the good so your older children or toddler know that they are on the right track when interacting with the baby.

The heartbreak of baby loss

I want to talk about baby loss here, which I know first-hand throws a dark shade on every subsequent pregnancy, and an anxiety over every moment of the last trimester until the newborn arrives safely. I'm sorry if this triggers any of you, but I feel women should share their stories – the heartbreak, the agony, the guilt – so we can rebuild together, knowing we are not alone.

In my pregnancy before Wolfie, when I started spotting, I rushed for a scan and was relieved to see the baby wiggling. But then as the days continued, my bleeding got heavier and heavier, and when I went for a second scan – although there was still a heartbeat – when the technician pulled out the vaginal ultrasound wand and it was covered in blood, I knew it wasn't normal. Still, the doctor insisted the heartbeat was healthy and strong, so we had an early celebration, announcing our news to our families, and started daydreaming about names as all expectant happy parents-to-be tend to do.

But a few weeks later, the bleeding started again and just wouldn't stop. I had a third scan, and when the technician looked at us sadly and said, 'I'm sorry, I can't hear a heartbeat,' I burst into tears. All I remember is Max grabbing my hand and holding it tightly. We headed to my gynaecologist who suggested a D&C (dilation and curettage), in case I got a blood infection, but we were supposed to be going on holiday with my brother to Corfu the next day and we really wanted to go, especially then, to escape for a bit. We went home, in a daze, not knowing what was happening, grief-stricken and not really knowing what to do. Shortly afterwards, I started to bleed. I ran upstairs and sat on the loo, crying my eyes out, Max hovering and not really knowing how to help. I saw a tiny little thing in the loo. We sent a photo to a doctor friend, who confirmed it was the foetus. We held hands and cried together again, but I also felt some sense of relief because it was a potential threat to my health if I continued to carry the foetus.

BEING POSITIVE AFTER BABY LOSS

DR NIHARA KRAUSE, CONSULTANT
CLINICAL PSYCHOLOGIST

The loss of a pregnancy before 20 weeks or miscarriage is an emotional life experience. Surprisingly common, but often not acknowledged for the devastating feelings encountered, miscarriage encapsulates not only all the different stages of grief but also initiates feelings of guilt, lack of confidence and worry about another pregnancy. While no 'one size fits all' in dealing with any emotional experience, here are five general tips that may help.

1. **Acknowledge what's individual to you about this experience and deal with each of these elements.** In general, there are two main factors relating to the pregnancy: previous history of pregnancies and miscarriages, and the situation surrounding the pregnancy (for example, long awaited, hard to conceive); and the circumstances surrounding the miscarriage, such as at what stage of pregnancy the miscarriage occurs. And then the factors relating to the individuals involved will also play a part. Is there, for example, a history of loss for either parent? How loss has been experienced, the mental health of either parent, both pre- and post-pregnancy, the nature and strength of the relationship, the amount of stress the person was under at the time of miscarriage are just some factors to consider.

2. **Permit yourself space and time to grieve. Choose how you would like to do this.** For some, grieving is a very private experience. In these instances, you may like to journal how you feel, do things you find comforting, share with a person you trust. For others, it might be seeking the comfort and connection of a group who have similar experiences or seeking professional support.

3. **Permit healing.** This might be about taking on a new challenge, building on strength and health, leaving aside the punitive voice of guilt by practising self-compassion, or connecting with a partner and exploring whether you are ready or want to try again.

4. **Trying again?** While fears of another miscarriage are common, the reality is that most women will have healthy pregnancies following a miscarriage. Talk to health professionals about your fears and focus on positive messages, do things that empower you, work on reducing stress, see the best in yourself (and note these things down, so that when negativity or guilt gets you down, you can remind yourself), push past obstacles by looking at the benefit that lies beyond them and by resolving them.

5. **See a specialist mental health professional** who can support you in making change.

Talk to health professionals about your
fears and focus on positive messages.

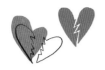

The next morning, we took the flight to Corfu, which might sound shocking but we really needed something positive to focus on, to get us out of our heads . . . which turned out to be impossible because my sister-in-law Lizzie was about to announce the joyous news that she was pregnant on that trip. We were trying to get pregnant at the same time, to raise cousins of the same age, and of course I was happy for her, but it felt like a blow. As soon as I found myself alone, I cried so hard in my bedroom – happy for her, but sad for me and the dream of same-age cousins that wouldn't be. For the rest of the holiday, Lizzie tried so hard not to be excited in front of me, bless her, but the tiniest things would happen – like during one ride on a speedboat, she instinctively clutched hold of her belly as we bumped along the waves. I was heartbroken . . . but hopeful.

And luckily, I got pregnant quite quickly again afterwards with Wolfie. I didn't feel ready to share the story of my miscarriage in public until I was past 12 weeks with him. I didn't want any more pain, or questions, or to feel people were watching my every move and studying my stomach until I felt positive enough. It felt right to post about my experience during Miscarriage Awareness Week, and so many people got in touch to thank me for talking about it. It's still quite taboo and women can feel alone. I don't think you can understand what it's like to go through a miscarriage unless you've gone through one yourself. And how long it takes for your body to realise it's not pregnant any more, and for your hormones and emotions to return to normal. You are a mess. Your body is still changing, but not growing a new life any more. It's a heartbreaking experience I will always remember.

That experience meant that although we were so happy to be pregnant again, we could never relax, or enjoy the scans, or plan too much. I was terrified the whole time. Every time I went to the loo and wiped, I'd be scared of seeing blood. But we moved on as best we could. Many people who have miscarriages don't tell people until the last trimester, in case the same thing happens again, but personally, I was glad people knew we were pregnant when we lost the baby – it meant they could help and support us, but everyone is different and we must be understanding.

BEING READY TO TRY
AGAIN AFTER MISCARRIAGE

ZOE CLARK-COATES MBE, GRIEF EXPERT AND
AUTHOR OF *SAYING GOODBYE, THE BABY LOSS
GUIDE* AND *PREGNANCY AFTER LOSS*

Trying for a baby after baby loss is such a hard decision for some people and a foregone conclusion for others. Often, I get asked if one can ever feel truly ready to try again, and I am not sure you can. The majority of people will be riddled with anxiety, and what makes people try again is that their fear of not having a child to raise is greater than their fear of encountering further loss. My fourth book *Pregnancy After Loss* helps guide you through this stage in your life, and it is packed with advice and professional support. My top suggestions include talking about your fears and worries – denying your feelings and not allowing your thoughts and concerns to be addressed can actually make them grow, so make space and time to process how you feel. Speak with your GP or medical team and ask them for advice and tips. Some useful questions to ask are: Could I be put on any drugs that might help? What vitamins should I be taking? Could they offer any tests to rule out issues – e.g., blood tests or scans? Am I physically ready to carry a baby? Try not to overthink the process of trying for a baby. There are so many tips on how best to conceive and when to try during the month. While some of this advice is helpful, it can also become all-consuming. If sex starts to be only about baby making, it can damage a relationship and can certainly affect the intimacy between you and your partner. Keep talking as a couple. The better you communicate, the easier everything will be and feel.

Give yourself time to recover emotionally if you feel you need it. We are always told to ensure we are physically ready, but it is just as important to feel mentally ready for another pregnancy, or even emotionally ready to try to get pregnant. I always advise people not to wait until they feel ready to lose again. Who would ever feel ready to lose another baby? It is like asking someone to wait to feel ready to be pushed off the edge of a cliff. When you enter a new pregnancy, you do so with the belief that all will be different this time, and you can only do this if you have faith things will be okay, and while some may feel this is naive, I believe it's holding on to hope with two hands. If you are blessed to get pregnant, consider telling people as soon as possible. The more people who know about your pregnancy, the more support you will be offered from those around you.

———

If sex starts to be only about baby making, it can damage a relationship and can certainly affect the intimacy between you and your partner. Keep talking as a couple. The better you communicate, the easier everything will be and feel.

———

Body positivity before baby

Particularly after baby loss, or just when pregnant for the first time, people are tempted to wrap themselves in cotton wool – and one way they do this is to stop exercising. Do what you want, I say! As long as it is safe to do so, of course. Do whatever makes you *you* – a happy, calm, healthy version of you. When I was pregnant with Wolfie I had previous experience of how my body was pregnant, so I did a little more exercise and ate a little healthier than I had done when I was pregnant with India so I could stay strong, until the last trimester. Max loves his food, eating is a real pleasure for both of us, and by the end of my pregnancy we were ordering in lots of delicious takeaways because I was tired and heavy, and to be honest thought what's the point of restricting myself now when I'm shaped like a beach ball anyway?

My saving grace was that towards the end of a pregnancy, when the baby is so big, you can't stuff much in your tummy anyway. And I was too hot to indulge too badly. It was a sweaty June and I just wanted to get the baby out! I had weird joint issues and was in quite a lot of pain and couldn't move my limbs very well, and I always needed a wee, so I couldn't sleep, which combined made me too tired to exercise too much – and that was fine. You have to listen to your body. Rest if you need to, work out if you'd like to. But do remember that old wives' tale of eating for two is total bollocks. Max definitely ate for two during my pregnancy but luckily, I refrained, well, to a degree (if I ignore the mass waffle consumption), which did make it easier to get back to my normal weight quicker after giving birth to Wolfie than it had with India, when I was naive about how my habits while pregnant would affect my postnatal body.

TOP FIVE TIPS FOR PRENATAL EXERCISE

ZOE ROBSON, FOUNDER OF FIT MUMS BERKSHIRE

1. Keep well hydrated and ensure you refuel your body well after exercise. This can help avoid any dizziness or nausea which can happen if you have not eaten or had enough fluids. If you do suffer with pregnancy heartburn/acid reflux, be mindful to wait 30 minutes or so after eating before exercising to avoid any discomfort.

2. It is safe to continue with cardiovascular exercises such as running, cycling and circuit training, but do not push yourself to the point of exhaustion. You shouldn't be so out of breath you are unable to speak while exercising. If you are unable to speak at any point this is a sign you need to scale back. Work to a max 7 out of 10 on the exertion scale.

3. Make sure you include pelvic floor exercises daily, ideally performing these three times a day. You want to ensure you practise both quick squeeze and releases (x10) and longer 10-second holds (x10) each time. I recommend downloading the NHS Squeezy app for helpful timers and daily reminders. If you have any pelvic floor dysfunction or pain it is worth seeing a women's health physio during your second or third trimester.

4. Work to 70–80 per cent of what you did before you were pregnant in terms of weight and the number of reps, for example, if you used to squat 15kg for 20 reps perhaps drop down to 10kg for 15 reps. It's likely by your third trimester you will need to make further modifications. When exercising be sure to focus on maintaining good posture, technique and breath control.

5. Allocate some time each week to stretch and relax. During pregnancy we want to maintain strength to support the postural changes but also have flexibility and mobility ready for the challenges of labour and prepare for postnatal recovery. In particular during pregnancy working on hip-opening poses and releases for your back will be really beneficial. Regular mobility exercises can help decrease symptoms of pelvic girdle pain and ease lower back pain which are common complaints during pregnancy.

Baby-proofing your life

I wasn't the best at doing the sensible, logistical part of baby-proofing – like installing stairgates, which I must do soon because Wolfie has started trying to throw himself down them three times a day, or buying those things you plug in electric sockets, or moving everything fragile or precious out of the way of baby hands. I did enjoy the most fun things like getting the nursery ready, setting myself little goals to achieve in those last three months of pregnancy like picking out wallpaper for his room and choosing a buggy. Spending your last baby-free weekends together with your partner doing that sort of thing is bonding and special; and I suggest not leaving it until the last minute in case the baby comes early, use the whole three months of the last trimester. On that note, get yourselves a lovely date night in a month before your due date because who knows when you'll next fancy a date night, or have the energy or willing help to go on one. And don't leave packing your hospital bag until the last minute either. You don't want to be caught without your big knickers or nipple cream. Checklists are your friend in these last few, hectic months of baby waiting.

Baby showers

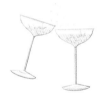

A friend threw me a shower when I was pregnant with Wolfie, and it turned into quite a big celebration, and it was really lovely. I know people can be funny about these celebrations because they feel a bit smug and American, especially when it's not your first baby, but when you make them personal and have games, they're fun, and life is hard so why not find happiness where possible.

DON'T FORGET BABY DADDIES

When I was pregnant with Wolfie, it was important for me to remember that although it was my second baby, it was Max's first. And your partner should be involved more in every pregnancy, the good and bad bits. All they get traditionally is a pint of beer to wet the baby's head the day it arrives, which is daft – you'll want your partner with you that day – so get it out of the way before! Max loved the shower. His friends got him some gifts and talked baby stuff. Mentally, becoming a parent is a big deal for your partner, too, and they likely worry more about being a good parent and provider than they probably let on. Often, they feel helpless – especially during labour when their partner is in pain and they can't help. They hate feeling useless, don't they? The good ones. It's important to make them feel a part of the process.

Preparing your partner in the last trimester

I think it's really important to have conversations with your partner before the baby arrives to work out a few rules. Don't let parenting creep up on you! Before you know it, you'll be screaming and squabbling and ultimately hating each other. Things can get nasty quickly when you're both tired and unsure of your roles and feeling lost. Because we had these chats in advance, we agreed that I would do the night shifts with Wolfie because Max had to still get up for work. He was really grateful, and it was my idea so I couldn't silently seethe with resentment. He'd pull his weight in other

STAYING CALM AS YOU PLAN FOR BABY

ANGY TSAFOS, LIFE AND MINDSET COACH,
ENERGY WORKER AND EFT PRACTITIONER

As a mother there is always so much to do. The list becomes never ending when you add to it the role of a loving wife/partner, domestic goddess, successful worker, caring daughter, supportive friend, etc. It's so easy to feel overwhelmed and unsure of where to begin. Firstly, I want to start by saying that this is completely natural and that there is nothing wrong with you. I have often found myself in a bit of a tangle, ready to give up, when I think of the sheer amount that needs to be done (in the last trimester).

My first suggestion is to make a list of all the things that need doing. Write it all down so you no longer let it all swirl in your head. Then pick the first task that appeals to you and that is the easiest to tick off. Focus on one thing at a time. Every time your mind wanders, take a deep breath – the biggest, longest belly breath and exhale through pursed lips. This will activate your parasympathetic system and help you find calm. Speak kindly to yourself by saying, 'It's okay, I know that there is a lot to do. I have my list and I am working my way through everything. I am doing my best. I am okay.' And breathe. If a task feels too big, then break it down to smaller more achievable tasks and chip at it in that way. Remember that you do not need to tackle everything at once. Often overwhelm shows up when we think of everything that needs to be done as a whole.

Do reach out and ask for help whenever you need it. There is no shame in saying that you cannot do it all. Your sanity and wellbeing are far more precious than proving that you are a superwoman who, by the way, doesn't exist! Besides, remember that you look after others best when you look after yourself first. Giving from an empty cup leads to burnout and resentment.

So, my final tip is to nurture yourself. When you are feeling overwhelmed, take a break and ask yourself, 'What would make me feel better right now? What support do I need?' It could be a nice cup of tea, a nice walk outside. Whatever it is that your heart is whispering to you, listen to it and give yourself that moment. It will help recharge your energy and your motivation to tackle your list. And remember to celebrate yourself as you tick tasks off your list.

THE MOST IMPORTANT THING YOU

CAN DO IN THE LAST TRIMESTER

KATE BALL, MUM OF SIX (INCLUDING TWO SETS OF
TWINS!) AND FOUNDER OF MINI FIRST AID

When we get ready for the baby to arrive, we often focus on the softer side: the nursery, the change bag, the pram, the first outfit. Why not? Having a baby is an exciting time. We then start to think about the birth, how we want things to go and how we plan to feed our baby. It is hard not to feel nervous as a new parent. Everything is unknown. At Mini First Aid we cannot give you all the magic answers about getting your baby to sleep through the night, but we can help you to think about practically equipping yourself for the baby, and to think about first aid. Attend a baby first aid class. Knowing what to do in an emergency could literally save a life. Ask the adults (grandparents and carers) who will be spending time with your baby to also attend a first aid class and don't forget siblings can attend first aid classes designed for children.

Make sure you have a first aid kit in your change bag or under your pram and another located at home in the room you spend most of your time in. Make sure that everyone knows where the first aid kit is kept and replenish supplies regularly. Find out which neighbours are at home at particular times of day, so that if you ever need emergency help, you know who you can call on. Make sure you know where your nearest Paediatric A & E is located (not all hospitals have one).

areas – cooking dinner or taking the children out for walks. Use the last trimester to go to prenatal baby classes together so you can both hear what to expect and meet other people who are about to land in the same new world as you. And in a world where everything, the good and the bad, is placed on the pregnant mum, remember your partner is having a baby too – it's a big deal for both of you. Include them or they might wind up feeling resentful towards you or the baby. You have to be a team.

Another last trimester?

Max would like two more children, I'd like one more, so that's still to be negotiated . . . I'm not going to rush anything though. I already feel very lucky to have two healthy children and a wonderful partner. It's funny how my life has really changed in the last five years. I was quite content on my own with India, the two of us against the world, a girl gang. I didn't want to rock the boat or upset anyone; I didn't want to lose any more time with my daughter. And then my mummy persuaded me to drive to my friend's thirtieth at Soho Farmhouse that Sunday, to be young and fun for a few hours . . . and there, at the party next door, was Max . . . and we fell in love, and then Wolfie arrived . . . and that was the making of us – against any odds I had been unconsciously waging against myself.

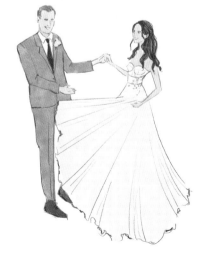

CHAPTER TWO

The First Month with a New Baby

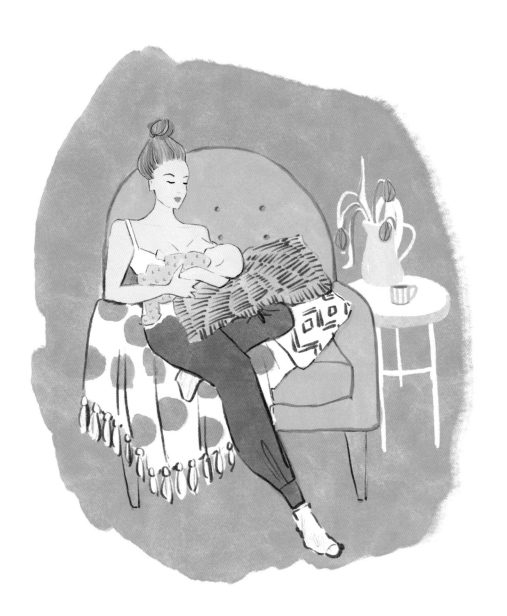

Let's admit it's scary when you first find yourself home alone with a baby, after being at hospital surrounded by experts, or at home wrapped up in the bubble of family, friends, doulas and midwives. And then suddenly – at least, sometimes – it's just you and baby, the most precious thing you've ever held, alone. That's a pressure. I know I was like, 'What the hell do I do now?' It's the best feeling in the world, but also the moment you have to step up. This gorgeous little thing needs you.

I brought India home on my twenty-seventh birthday. My mummy and sister had done an excellent job of making my flat as welcoming as possible for us to return to – despite the building mess – switching the lamps on, putting up cards and buying yummy treats. They settled us in and left – and I felt happy at first. It didn't hit me, the magnitude of motherhood, until I was trying to breastfeed India a few nights later, when we had some friends over to make dinner for us. She wouldn't settle, wouldn't feed, and I felt this pressure to be social – to still be *me* – but she wouldn't stop crying, and so I started crying. I did what I often did in that first month of motherhood:

I FaceTimed my mum, who was with my sister, who burst out laughing. 'Chill out and stop being so hard on yourself. Give her a bottle. Give her formula. Have a glass of wine,' they said. So, I did – and she slept really well, and I reclaimed some of my sanity.

We got into a groove for the rest of the first month after that moment, setting up a sweet little routine, me snacking on toast and tea, India having a bottle. The only other scary thing was putting her in a baby car seat and driving on my own for the first time. And of course, I had a camera crew filming my every move. I couldn't work the bloody thing out for ages – the buckles, the straps. And then once she was securely in, I would get followed by paparazzi. I remember during that first month, I drove us to the country to see a friend who was visiting from Italy, trailed the whole time by photographers – three or four cars – who were jumping red lights, chasing me. I was scared, and more so because I had this tiny baby to take care of. They followed me off the motorway and down some twisty, one-lane country roads. When I finally reached my friend, who had just had a baby the week before and answered the front door practically with her boobs hanging out, I was a mess and she was confused. 'What the hell is going on?' I remember her saying, as I collapsed into her home. 'Who have you brought with you?' They followed me right to her house!

That was the worst of it, but it was exciting too – and most of the time I didn't mind being a new mum in the public eye. I had a lot of interaction with followers on social media that was largely positive and encouraging, and it gave me a platform to share my experiences. I look back at the footage now and can't believe how unkempt I look – my hair extensions had become matted. I was so exhausted, I didn't wear an ounce of make-up, and lived in tracksuits. I mean, I looked like I smelt! I've watched a few people in the industry go through that first month of motherhood since I did, with their impeccable clothes, hair and make-up, and call bullshit. The first photo the press got of me post-India was in the street, hair in a messy topknot, probably with some spit-up on me, not even wearing sunglasses . . . and that's the reality of that first month of motherhood. Don't worry about it. Self-compassion is needed now more than ever.

A happy hibernation

The other reality uncovered during that first month is that you can stop the world and cocoon for a little bit, people expect it of you. This little person needs you and doesn't understand work–life balance, to-do lists or timelines. I headed to Sussex with Mummy for most of the month, got out of the paddling pool, laid India down in the shade on a sheepskin rug, and old friends came to meet her. I got to recreate this for Wolfie's first month too – but this time in that extra sweet space of being a family with Max and India. We had the most gorgeous bubble I will always be grateful for – again with a paddling pool, and this time a bubble machine to entertain India as we whiled away the afternoons. We were just so happy together. I remember a moment as clearly as anything: both my children had fallen asleep on me, snuggled and content, after a long day of fresh air and sunshine, and I knew then that life couldn't get any better. I think I'm very lucky that I've had two summer babies, having them in the garden with no clothes on, and going for lovely long walks in the pram and picnics in the park. Things must be harder for you mums who have winter babies, with the chilly, dark mornings and the array of colds and viruses going around. I'm all for a nestle down in front of a log fire, without feeling guilty for hibernating and staying indoors, but I think summer makes that initial plunge into motherhood easier.

LEARNING SELF-COMPASSION

ANGY TSAFOS, LIFE AND MINDSET COACH,
ENERGY WORKER AND EFT PRACTITIONER

Learning to be kind to myself has been a lifelong journey. It's so easy to be overly critical of oneself, especially when social media is showing us how perfect everyone else seems to be. But let me tell you this: everyone has an inner mean girl. She has the bad habit of popping up every time we make mistakes, doubt ourselves, feel a bit low or are outside of our comfort zone trying something new. She is the faithful companion that we wish we did not have because let's face it, she does a stellar job at making us feel miserable. Weirdly though, if we delve a little bit deeper, we will find that she is only trying to protect us from getting hurt. Unfortunately, if we do listen to her, we stay small and nothing we ever do is good enough.

MISTAKES MAKE YOU A BETTER PERSON. The first thing to remember is that everyone makes mistakes. We may feel embarrassed, ashamed or feel like we are the worst mother on earth. However, mistakes make us stronger and wiser. Turn these into a learning opportunity. Ask yourself – what have I learned? What will I do next time? And then move on. There is no need to dwell on it because you have now identified your learning and are equipped for the future.

PRACTISE TREATING YOURSELF WITH COMPASSION. If this does not come easily to you or you are struggling to quieten that inner critic, then imagine that your best friend or your child came to you and shared these terrible comments. What would you say to them to lift them up and support them? What words of encouragement are needed right now? Do not hesitate to tell yourself these words. Have trust – it gets easier the more you practise this. The first step is to recognise that your inner mean girl is here and that she is the one talking – this is not the real you. Giving her a name (mine is 'Mildred') is a great way to distance yourself from her and see her as the eternal pessimist who brings you down with their negativity. So when Mildred starts listing all the things that you did wrong or would not be able to do, greet her and thank her for caring but then promptly ask her to shut up and go sit in the corner.

CHANGE MILDRED'S NEGATIVE COMMENTS INTO SOMETHING POSITIVE.
Change 'You don't know what you are doing. You are such an idiot – just
give up now' to 'I have never done this before, so it's okay that it's taking me
longer to complete. I am learning and I am doing the best I can. It will get
better. I can do this!' Affirmations are also perfect if you need a boost and are
a great way to create new positive neural pathways.

DO NOT ACT ON WHAT SHE TELLS YOU TO DO. Her advice is very rarely
the right kind to take. Gently ask her to go sit in the corner, and distract
yourself by doing something else or focusing on the task at hand by being
mindful. For example, notice the colours around you, pay attention to how
your legs feel against your seat. Your inner mean girl is misguided but well
meaning. She is trying to prevent you from doing something that she fears
will make you look bad or to simply provoke a reaction despite your better
judgement. Unfortunately, at some point in your life, your inner mean girl
has learned from past experience (maybe as a result of an exchange with a
parent, a teacher or a meanie at school) that by nagging or being harsh, she
will obtain the right reaction that will keep you safe. So, if you are feeling
game and strong, go ahead and ask your inner critic why she is saying these
things to you. What is she hoping to achieve? What is she afraid of if she
stops talking to you like that? Once you have the answer, you can take the
appropriate steps to calm her or even give yourself the moral support you
need to move forwards.

Remember that your inner mean girl will always be present in some way
or another because we are all human. When you hear her whispering or
shouting in your ears, don't lose heart but apply the techniques you have
learned. Practice makes perfect – so keep going even when it feels tough!

LEARNING TO GET ALONG TOGETHER

What advice would I give for making it through that nerve-wracking first month? Be confident in your own abilities. Chill out, because if you're tense your baby could pick up on it. I'd leave India safely strapped into her chair and take a shower. I'd let her cry for a minute before rushing to her side in a panic. If your baby is safe, try not to overly worry. I had friends worrying about the exact temperature of their baby's milk, and then because they were so particular, the baby would be programmed to scream if it didn't arrive just as they expected. I didn't start any of that. It would turn the child into a fussy nightmare!

So that's my main piece of advice: be careful what routines you start at the very beginning . . . because you'll have to keep them going the whole time. Think about what works for the baby *and* you. Consider carefully what you will be able to continue. I didn't have blackout blinds or a white noise sound machine because I didn't want to get into the habit of me or her not being able to live without them when we travelled. I've got friends that have to bring the whole nursery with them every time they leave the house for the night, and I can't deal with that hassle and fuss. I've got friends who got their babies so used to sleeping in a crib that they refuse to nap in the car or in their buggy, really restricting what their parents are free to do. I know babies who demand silence at bedtime, whereas from day one I'd place India in her bassinet and keep her with me when I had friends over for dinner, so she can sleep anywhere. Don't start anything you don't want to commit to. You can't spoil your baby – love your baby, hug your baby, talk to your baby . . . but remember they do need to fit in around your life too, and buying all the extra paraphernalia isn't proof of love. It's just stuff.

YOUR POST-BABY BODY

REBECCA STEVENS, NUTRITIONIST

Pregnancy affects the physical appearance of our postnatal bodies – there's stretch marks, abdominal muscle separation and weight gain. While the changes are all a normal part of growing a baby, they can leave you feeling like your body is no longer your own. On top of this, there is also the added pressure of feeling like you should 'bounce back' as quickly as those on social media or, closer to home, your new mum friend down the road. According to a UK study, 73 per cent of women weighed more than their pre-pregnancy weight at six months postpartum (Hollis et al., 2017). So, in other words, just 1 in 4 women had lost their pregnancy weight. If you are struggling, you are most definitely not alone and understanding the factors working against you in this phase of life can hopefully help you to be a little kinder to yourself.

Try to remember that your recovery journey is a very personal and unique experience. While it can be all too easy to compare yourself to others on the same journey, try to avoid this. Congratulate your body on what an incredible job it has just performed. Think about all the different factors that influence your recovery, e.g., size of your baby, position of your baby in the womb, the amount of weight gained in pregnancy, how well your baby does or doesn't sleep, how much help you have at home, the number of children you have, the natural elasticity of the skin, etc.

While it is advisable to lose the weight gained in pregnancy to support your own health and to begin any subsequent pregnancies at a healthy weight for your body, losing this weight needs to happen in the right way, which isn't as quickly as possible, as this isn't best for your body or the baby that you are now caring for. Try to be kind to yourself and remember that time frames to return to your pre-pregnancy weight will be different for everyone.

Research shows that reduced sleep duration, which all new mums experience, has an impact on our food choices and dietary habits. You crave certain foods when tired, particularly of the sugary kind. With all stages of life, we are aiming for balance within our diets so if you fancy the less healthy snack options don't restrict yourself completely. If you are breastfeeding, this can have an impact on your food choices and dietary habits because it can be difficult to prepare the food you'd like to eat, at the time you'd like to eat it. Breastfeeding requires extra calories (around 500kcal/day) so you will need to eat more to support your body to make the breast milk. Hence why trying to lose the weight in the early postnatal phase shouldn't be the priority. Being a mum of a newborn is a 24/7 role. Your nutrition, or what you eat in this phase of life, plays an important role in your overall health. But it can be incredibly difficult to eat well with all the extra demands on your time. If you choose to breastfeed, you'll also need to be eating more to provide your body with the energy to produce the milk.

As a nutritionist and mum of three, I'm often asked what new mums should be snacking on. The answer is to aim for snacks that are nutrient-dense so that they not only fill you up but provide other nutritional benefits. This doesn't mean you can't have some cake or similar when you feel like some; this is not the time to be restrictive. Look for healthy snacks that are tasty, filling, nutritious and easy to prepare – and can be easily thrown in the bottom of a buggy or nappy bag. I love hummus with pitta bread and crudités, bananas, trail mix, nuts or nut butter on toast, edamame beans – from the soya family, these beans are a good protein source and include magnesium, iron and fibre. Plain Greek yogurt is another good protein source, add berries and a sprinkle of mixed seeds for extra vitamins, fibre and antioxidants. Boiled eggs – admittedly not everyone's favourite but these are handy little snacks and can be boiled earlier in the day and eaten when you fancy; oat cakes provide energy and if you add cheese, you get protein and calcium. Last but not least, energy balls are great, too – there are a range of these in the shops these days so try out a few and select your favourite.

Also don't forget to stay hydrated, your body needs extra water when breastfeeding and it is very easy to become dehydrated. Don't wait for those dehydration headaches to set in before reaching for some water or other drink of your choice.

The shock of motherhood

I didn't go through the identity crisis or the post-baby blues that many women go through in that first month; for me, motherhood felt natural. I've seen some very dear friends struggle though, and I always tell them, 'I know you feel vulnerable or silly reaching out to people you trust, but you must – they can help you.' Tell at least one person how you're feeling. Communicating is crucial. There are lots of helplines out there. Not everyone feels the rush of love when they hold their baby for the first time. You're not weird. You're not alone. You're not evil. Your body and your brain have gone through a lot. I know a few new mothers who have struggled with intrusive thoughts. Some have had them so badly that they've been driving along with the baby screaming in the back and considered what a relief it would be to turn the wheel and crash into a wall, ending the noise and the self-loathing. You're not thinking rationally because of the new, extreme pressures you are under. These are unwanted, intrusive thoughts. It's not what you really want to do, and you need to know that these thoughts are common, and you can talk to people who understand. We discuss this at Bloss; clearing up misinformation and those elements of mothering that are difficult to comprehend or come to terms with. A friend, who had a baby three weeks before I had India,

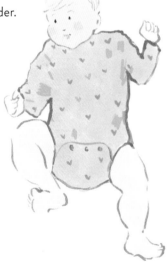

put me in this mommy group called Wild Mamas. The other women were all a bit older and were really bloody cool. We're still bonded as a group. There's no jealousy. There's no bitchiness. I met Steph, my business partner, there ... and Bloss grew from our real-life friendship and need for a wise, strong community, which is so important – particularly at the beginning of your life as a mum. Information is all in one place, from conception to teenage tantrums, made clear by experts we've vetted and trust.

As I grew as a mummy, with India and Bloss, I appreciated another important rule to set from the beginning: you can say no. To people popping over all the time, to people overstaying their welcome, to people demanding too much of you, or expecting you to follow their advice. This is about you and the baby bonding. Shut the door, switch off your phone, come off social media, yawn and ask people to leave. Allow good friends and family to visit but set a time limit. Warn them not to expect to be fed. It's nice to have company sometimes, but you also have to protect your cocoon and your sleep quota.

This is about you and the baby bonding. Shut the door, switch off your phone, come off social media, yawn and ask people to leave.

SAFELY HANDLING SLEEP

WITH A NEWBORN

KATE BALL, FOUNDER OF MINI FIRST AID

Inevitable sleep deprivation in parents can compromise their ability to follow safer sleep guidelines for their children, resulting in an increased risk of sudden infant death syndrome (SIDS). On average, parents get less than 59 per cent of the recommended 8 hours of sleep a night in the first 12 months after having a baby, according to a recent study by sleep technology brand Simba, which can have a serious impact on a parent's ability to function both mentally and physically. Mini First Aid looks at the effects of sleep deprivation, and how, despite the general befuddlement this results in, we as parents can still help our babies sleep safely.

Sleep deprivation is something new parents often joke about, but it's no laughing matter. A significant lack of sleep can start to affect your body in many ways and can make it much harder for us to think rationally and logically. Moodiness, forgetfulness, becoming accident prone and unable to concentrate – almost every parent has a story to tell about when they accidentally put the car keys in the freezer or left the house with their slippers on – we often accept as just part of the parenting journey.

However, sleep deprivation can have serious consequences when parents get tempted to compromise on the safer sleep guidelines 'just for one night' because they are so tired. The Lullaby Trust want to raise awareness of the importance of always following the safer sleep guidelines for your little ones, even when you are at your most tired, to reduce the risk of sudden infant death syndrome (SIDS). Prepare your baby's safe sleep space in advance before you give birth. This means as soon as your baby is born you can hit the ground running and won't need to think about whether the sleep environment is safe alongside everything else you will be thinking about in those early days. Think about a short 'safer sleep routine' that you could follow before every nap or night time. For example, check the temperature of the room, get baby dressed, take everything out of the sleep space, give baby their dummy and lay baby down on their back. If you repeat these things in the same order every time, then it will become a habit and help ensure your baby sleeps safely at every nap.

Ask your partner, a friend or a family member to sit with the baby or take them out for a walk while you catch up on some shut-eye and recuperate. Share the Lullaby Trust safer sleep guidelines with anyone who will have responsibility for your little one, whether that's your partner, grandparents, a child minder or your wider family and friends. The more you make people aware of them, the more likely they are to follow them, which will help your baby sleep safer.

Sleep is precious so take any chance you can get, forget about stacking the dishwasher when baby is napping and lay down yourself for some rest, even if you can't nap, just try to take a break. If you are breastfeeding, then you might like to try expressing some milk once you and your baby have established breastfeeding, so your partner could take over one of the night feeds and you can sleep for longer. You and your partner could make a 'lie-in plan' so you can take it in turns to get up with the children in the morning so that the other one can sleep in and rest uninterrupted. Sleep deprivation can sometimes (ironically) make it difficult to fall asleep when your head finally touches the pillow. Children and adults alike can suffer from being 'overtired' which makes it hard to switch off. If this happens to you, then you might like to try taking a bath, reading a book or switching off any electronic devices like your mobile phone at least 30 minutes before bedtime to give your brain a chance to switch off.

_____

Sleep is precious so take any chance you can get.

_____

The first month of fatherhood

I never had any worries about how Max would be as a dad to a newborn because I'd already seen him in action with India from when she was a toddler. He's very level-headed, a cool dude whose opinions I really respect. If anything, he became an even better dad to India when Wolfie came along, as if proving to us all that he loved India unconditionally. Equally. He'd take her for daddy dates while I was at home with the baby, making sure she never felt ignored or excluded. We were a team from the first day. It makes me feel fuzzy just thinking about those first few weeks as a family of four. We bought India a little scooter and ventured up to the village, where she'd proudly introduce her baby brother to everyone we bumped into.

You do have to remember, even when you're bone tired and resentful that your partner gets to leave the house to go to work each day, that these first few weeks especially are about teamwork. Communicate clearly what you need. Don't let the niggles and annoyances build up. That's when the shouting starts. Your partner isn't psychic and will be having different worries or ideas to you. Understand that every couple gets stressed at this time. You're not doing something wrong. In fact, why people have a baby to fix a broken relationship is beyond me – I can't think of a quicker way for the wheels to come off a partnership than by adding a screaming, shitting newborn to the mix.

Looking after yourself

The rough times with a newborn for me were always in the night, or the morning after the night before when I was so tired, I could hardly think. If I don't get enough sleep, my anxiety gets quite bad. Therefore, as a mother, I've started to take better care of myself – and I urge you to, too. You have to be in the right headspace to parent; you must look after your own health. For me, especially with a tiny baby, it means having a shower, washing my hair, getting out into the fresh air, listening to music, and finding the joy in the little things. Remember to be grateful. Don't get upset that you're still going to be carrying a bit of extra weight, or that you're not going to get dressed up and look glamorous, or that your high heels are going to stay chucked in the back of the wardrobe for a bit longer. You made a human being, woman! Give yourself a break.

And if you're a woman who is chomping to get back in the gym because it makes you feel healthier and stronger, good for you. I'm the same. Just make sure you're ready. I got myself an internal examination to make sure everything was strong enough. And I remembered that there's no quick fix, but with determination you will start feeling yourself again before you know it. Remember that old-fashioned saying: nine months in, nine months out. That's the time frame you should give your body to return to how it was (well, almost, you might always have a saggier tummy and a saggier vag) if you want it to . . . nine months. That is where I am when I write this chapter. Wolfie is nine months old now, and the physical dust is settling. He's just started to sleep through the night, which means I can too. My energy is returning so I'm back to classes, and seeing a personal trainer, and Max and I go for long walks pushing Wolfie in his stroller, which keeps us healthy and doubles as a date, because we talk non-stop as we're striding along. Walking and talking is a good thing for couples actually – there's less pressure than if you've booked a babysitter, a table at a romantic restaurant, then you're sat opposite each other with one eye on the clock. Being out in nature makes us all feel calm – even Wolfie.

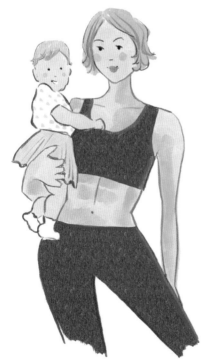

You have to be in the right headspace to parent; you must look after your own health.

WELLBEING IN

'THE FOURTH TRIMESTER'

DR ELIZABETH ALMAS, FUNCTIONAL MEDICINE DOCTOR

The fourth trimester begins and suddenly it is ALL about the baby! But what is the baby without you to be there, strong, positive and healthy, looking after it. Pregnancy depletes our bodies of 10 per cent of our most vital vitamins and minerals that we need to function optimally. We spend nine months nourishing and feeding the baby from our stores, leaving us with a hole to fill! Mineral loss, combined with the physiological stress of not sleeping and caring for a new life, can leave us feeling drained. Over time, it can have a big impact on our adrenal health, thyroid health and mental health. This is why hair mineral testing prior to pregnancy, during and after can be so incredibly important and informative as it shows us what we are missing and what to replenish, making it an individual, effective and targeted approach to quicker recovery.

For example, the stress on your body of pregnancy, birth and sleepless nights early on will hugely reduce your magnesium levels. Magnesium is essential for our mental wellbeing, it is required to make thyroid hormones that help keep us energised, it makes melatonin which we need for sleep and plays an important role in keeping our bowels moving in those early days! In fact, magnesium alone is responsible for over 600 enzymatic reactions in your body. Similarly, baby blues, postpartum depression and the more severe cases of postpartum psychosis can in fact be linked back to vitamin and mineral imbalances. For example, we are advised to avoid vitamin A in pregnancy due to toxicity to the foetus. However, to nourish the foetus requires huge amounts of vitamin A from the mother's stores and almost everyone we see is depleted in their third and fourth trimesters. This then leads to increased levels of unbound copper in the blood. It is not that we get too much copper, it is that we need vitamin A to use copper correctly and if we do not have enough, copper is left to roam free. This excess copper settles on the brain and can be the catalyst for post-baby blues and more.

The good thing is that supporting your wellbeing in pregnancy and after is easy if you know how. I recommend a few things to mothers to prepare for the fourth trimester:

1. Ideally get a hair mineral test three months before you try for a baby and replenish any deficits you have. Going into pregnancy strong is vital for how you feel after you've given birth.

2. In between any morning sickness, try to eat the rainbow for phytonutrients, lots of root vegetables to increase butyrate, which supports the gut where hormones are made, omega-3 fish oils for vitamin A, needed for your red blood cells, and eggs for choline, needed for the baby's brain health.

3. Take in 2.5–3 litres of mineral-rich hydration, including sparkling water, 150ml of coconut water combined with ½ teaspoon of rock salt, and 150ml orange juice daily.

4. At the start of the third trimester, do another hair mineral test to assess your mineral depletion and your thyroid and adrenal health. With the results in hand, start to nourish and supplement any minerals you are low in. Choose food first, supplements second. At this point, test your vitamin A levels; if they are low, eat whole food sources of vitamin A – liver is the most nourishing if you can stomach it! If not, take a whole food-derived beef liver supplement and get on the omega-3 fish oils daily.

5. Once you have delivered your baby, do not stop eating to get slim. Long term, eating more at this stage will allow your body to normalise quicker. You need nourishment to repair yourself and to support your thyroid and adrenals. If you eat too little, these glands slow down, making long-term weight loss and recovery incredibly difficult.

6. Get a final hair mineral test 4–6 months after the birth for a final insight into how your body has recovered and if there are any areas that you can work on specifically through diet or supplementation to restore yourself back to the level of vitality you deserve!

Becoming a new version of you

I did feel expectations coming at me when I first became a mum. Because I was on television and in *Made in Chelsea* specifically, a show known for its rich kids, I think people just expected me to have a full-time nanny and loads of help. I didn't have any of that. I didn't want it. I'd always wanted to be a mum and was happy to embrace this new part of my life. I was aware that some people wanted me to fail – even friends, who I obviously understand now were never *real* friends, just hangers-on who got their serotonin boosted when those around them suffered or struggled. These people can eat away at you. But whenever they made me second guess myself, I'd pull myself together and use my common sense: was I doing okay? Behaving well? Caring for my baby? Yes. I'd switch off the external noise as much as I could. This is hard to do in the first month when you're so tired and everything is changing, but I promise you so much comes back to common sense. Use the notes section at the back of this book to keep track of how you're feeling and what you hope to do to make you feel better. Often just writing things down gives you clarity. Make a list of people who make you feel good about yourself and your choices . . . and those who don't!

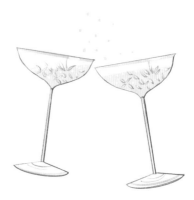

Luckily for me, these vampires were outweighed by the kind people who were – and are – rooting for me, and I'll never be able to show my appreciation enough. I still remember how happy people were for me, friends and strangers, when I met Max. I'd been a single mum for a while, so it really did seem like a happy ending, and I got lots of messages from other women on their own with young children who told me how I'd encouraged them to believe anything good can happen.

That's really my guide to the first month. Protect your peace. Enjoy your cocoon. Trust that even though you can't imagine ever feeling rested, sexy or clean again at the moment, this too shall pass. And really get into the mindset that even though you love this little creature more than anything – more than you love yourself – you're going to be together a long time, so set up a plan that works for both of you. They might be your world, but the world does not revolve around them. Besides, no one loves a spoiled, whiny kid who wants everything their own way. Those children don't get invited to birthday parties. Your biggest job as a parent is to raise a child who is adaptable, likeable and content in all manner of situations . . . and it's never too early to start.

———

Protect your peace. Enjoy your cocoon.

———

CHAPTER THREE

Co-parenting and Blended Families

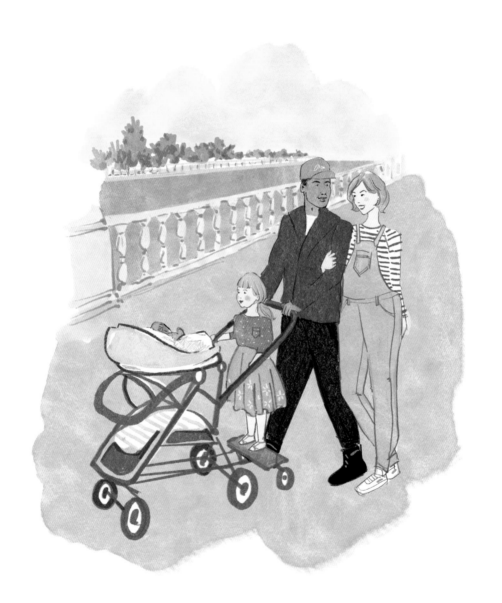

I remember the years my parents were breaking up very clearly; I remember the crying, the fighting, the choosing sides. It was an alien time for a pre-teen child to go through. I started counselling then and have never really stopped. Mummy and I moved away to Brighton, and I remember my dad being upset as our relationship fell apart because of the distance and because I was so close to my mum. It wasn't fair, in hindsight, because I'm sure he was trying his best. This hindsight has helped so much as I've navigated my own public break-up with India's dad.

Mummy became everything to me during these years of changes. I used to sleep in bed with her every single night without fail, even though I was too old. She was my mother, my saviour, my best friend, and I know she felt the same about me. We kept each other going with our inside jokes and closeness, which is sad to look back on now. There was too much pressure on us both to be each other's everything. But I needed her, and not only because she was my only constant parent, but because my school life was so bad. I was a country girl who'd been growing up in a lovely bubble one minute, then in a city school where the girls smoked, shagged and shoplifted the next. I'd dread going in every morning, crying so much at their cruel words that I wasn't able to sing the hymns in chapel. Confessing to Mummy what was going on, she promised to get her ducks in a row and get me back into the country as soon as she could. True to her word, we returned to a charming cottage in East Sussex, where she met a lovely man who became a father figure to me for a few years – and even better, he had two daughters who became like older sisters until they broke up some time later. It felt like after a few rough years of standing on a floor of smashed plates, we were finally able to put the china back up on the shelves.

My parents made a few parenting mistakes when they were going through their divorce that I didn't want to replicate. As an eleven- and twelve-year-old, I knew too much, the information I had was biased, and I hated seeing my mum so upset. I think Mummy shared too much, which wasn't particularly fair on me, and I'd have probably had a stronger relationship with my dad when I was a teenager if she hadn't treated me as a confidante. My father has since passed but I think my relationship with him would have been nicer if they'd hidden more from me.

Becoming a single mum

Obviously, with my history, I was scared of removing India from the stereotypical mum and dad at home life, but I knew I had to be strong and that it would be best for all three of us in the long run. My main concern was giving up time with her. She was so young when I split up with her father – barely one year old, still my baby – so being away from her was horrific. Each time she'd go I'd cry, and cry, and cry. The first time she knew she had to go off with him overnight, it felt like my heart was being torn out of my body. I just drove straight to my mum's and we went to the country. I knew I needed to distract myself and get out of London. Four years on, it doesn't get any easier. She's older so I'm able to explain to her that Mummy always comes back, and Mummy is never going anywhere. She is able to understand that now, whereas before, God knows what was going through her brain! The thought of it makes me feel sick to this day, that she could have possibly thought that she was being taken away and not coming back to me. I started a little routine to make us both feel better, slipping something small into her pocket or bag that she could look at and feel connected to me.

SHARING YOUR CHILD

Probably some of your exes assume the other parent is putting negative thoughts into their child's head about leaving them when the child shows signs of not wanting to go. It wasn't true in my case. It was awkward. I just wanted India to be happy, and I always remembered he was her father no matter what. Communication can be so difficult when there's hurt and resentment involved. If you're struggling to communicate – if you can't talk without fighting – then having a mediator can be super-helpful. Having a friend that can speak up for you calmly if you can't speak to each other, someone who isn't biased, someone who loves everyone involved, can stop custody situations from becoming atrocious. And think about getting a court order too if things become very difficult. Each party – both parents and child – needs to have boundaries, routines and arrangements that can be trusted and relied upon, and if it needs to be court ordered, to limit the muck ups, get lawyers involved. It stops difficult conversations or odd requests. Everyone knows where they are.

CALM CO-PARENTING

FOTOULLA MENIKOU, THE FRIENDLY FAMILY
LAWYER AND LEGAL EXPERT

Working out a contact schedule is a crucial aspect of successful co-parenting. Attending to the needs of your children first and foremost, is key to making a parenting schedule work. The schedule is also an important step in helping your children adjust to having divorced or separated parents. Try to consider as many eventualities as you can and be as specific as possible, to avoid potential conflict down the line. It's important to factor in things such as school events, medical appointments, holidays, meal times, extracurricular activities, bedtime routines, etc. This will help to craft a schedule that works best for your children and provide them with the consistency and stability they need. It will also help to minimise miscommunications between you and your co-parent, letting you each know your responsibilities within your respective households.

There may very well be instances where a co-parent has a job or other life variables which cannot easily be adjusted to enable a regular, consistent parenting schedule to be achieved. In these circumstances, communication and a degree of flexibility are crucial. If you are a parent who is not readily available to visit with your children or have overnight contact with them, then consider alternative options to help you maintain meaningful contact, such as video chat or instant messaging systems. If your children are old enough, do try to ascertain their wishes and work them into any contact schedule, wherever possible. It is also important to understand that as your children grow, a parenting schedule will need to evolve with them. This is why communication and flexibility are key, as is remembering that your children have a right to a relationship with both of their parents.

Things to avoid:

- **DON'T FOCUS ON CONVENIENCE:** As tempting as it may be, try to avoid creating a schedule which is convenient for you as a parent. The paramount consideration should always be to provide ongoing care and support for your children. This will undoubtedly require a healthy dose of compromise and some sacrifices along the way will be needed. Going into the process knowing this will help you to manage your own expectations and reduce irritations along the way.

- **DON'T THINK IN TERMS OF WINNING OR LOSING:** It can also be tempting to keep track of the sacrifices you are making in comparison to your co-parent, which will only breed animosity between you. Remember that the goal is to do what is best for your children, even if your co-parent appears to be less than co-operative. You will each be making sacrifices in different ways along your co-parenting journey.

- **DON'T ASSUME YOU'RE THE MORE QUALIFIED PARENT:** It is often the case that one parent will have more experience in dealing with specific routines, such as bedtime, bath time and school routines, but that doesn't necessarily mean that your co-parent cannot learn these skills too with a little help, guidance and encouragement.

Communication and flexibility are key, as is remembering that your children have a right to a relationship with both of their parents.

I suggest getting the outline of your co-parenting system sorted as soon as possible. You need to keep your weekends set in stone as much as you can, or you won't ever be able to plan anything – and we all need things to look forward to. Don't be unreasonable with requests, but don't be so flexible you don't know whether you're coming or going. Constant changes mean constant communication too, which can be draining. I try to keep things generic and amicable for India and constantly remind her that she is loved in both homes.

Bite your tongue when it comes to talking to or about your ex. However awful things get between adults, your child doesn't need to see it. However you're feeling about your child's father or mother, at the end of the day, they don't need to know the nitty-gritty stuff. They need to be kept as safe as possible, physically and mentally. If you must, share the truth when they're older and mature enough to understand it, not before.

THE GRANDPARENTS ARE GOOD

Try to maintain a healthy relationship with your former partner's parents, siblings and extended family. It will only benefit your child. You don't have to be in each other's pockets, but send Christmas cards, be civil. Your ex's mum will probably understand more about what you've been through with her child than anyone else – she knows them best, warts and all. Grandmas generally love their grandkid nearly as much as you do and have their best interests at heart.

However awful things get between adults, your child doesn't need to see it.

Judged as a single mum

I already knew I stood out as a young mum, but as a young *single* mum? I was expecting judgement but luckily the rude comments, if there were any, didn't make it back to me. I did feel like a failure, but that all came from within my own head – no one actually described me that way. Despite that, I still knew that India was the best thing to ever happen to me. I can't lie, it was tough at times being a single parent, but I still look at her and the time when it was just the two of us as the best gift ever. I wouldn't change a thing.

The only real judgement I feared was that of prospective dates. Who would want to date a single mum? Who would ever want to marry a twentysomething with a kid? Would I end up alone, dying in a room full of cats? I thought I'd be single for ever, so I wasn't looking for a relationship. Meeting Max was a wonderful shock, but I was scared to rock the boat at first. India and I had found a peaceful flow that I knew dating someone would disrupt. But I truly believe that everything happens for a reason, so although the timing might not have been ideal, I knew instantly there was something worth pursuing.

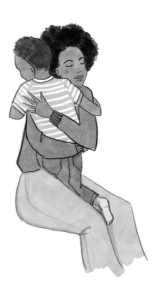

Introducing a new partner

India and I were set up as this safe little twosome, us girls against the world, when Max appeared. I was upfront with him about being a mother from our very first conversation. When he asked me what I did, I told him before anything else that I was India's mummy. He didn't bat an eyelid, which of course was so impressive. And shocking, really, because I was so nervous about how a man would take that news. When he asked me to go out for dinner with him, despite really liking him, I didn't really want to go – again, I was afraid of upsetting the status quo we had achieved, but Mummy told me not to be silly and to go . . . and it was the best date ever. I came away smiling, happy, it was the best feeling I've ever had after a first date. He was warm, open and honest and didn't make me feel like he just wanted to shag me. I knew it wasn't just a fling, even on the first date, and he knew and understood what a big step I was taking.

Our relationship developed naturally, easily. We got away on the weekends that India was at her father's, making amazing memories – which helped stop me from missing her enormously – and allowed us space to get to know each other. The moment he met her for the first time was casual – an accident actually! I'd had a minor prang in my car, nothing serious – but it had left a scratch – and when I sent him a photo, he said he'd be over in 5 minutes to help fix it. My first reaction was, 'Shit, no, I just picked up India from nursery,' but actually looking back it was probably a great first meeting because I couldn't overthink it. It was thrown at me. I wasn't just nervous about them meeting, but I was scared because it would be the first time that he saw the *real* me in my *real life*. Not dressed-up, fun, single Binky. I had to suddenly do the biggest shift – this was all or nothing.

He knocked on the door, I answered, and he walked in and smiled at India, knelt to get down on her level, said hi, and I was blown away by how calm it was. He checked out my car, then played with her for a bit, then we decided to go for a walk to the park with the dog, and I was pushing the pram with India in it, and it wasn't an issue. We were talking, and walking and laughing, and it felt right. Maybe that was the first moment we started making the us we are today. I remember thinking, 'I'm so freaking lucky because this is going to work,' and feeling so warm and wholesome.

On our first date he'd said to me, 'I know you're going to be the best mother to my children, because I'm lucky I already know that you're a great mum.' It was a risk for him to put himself out there like that but of course I loved it. I can sniff a wanker out a mile off these days, and I knew he wasn't just blowing smoke up my arse. I knew he meant it, and that he was naturally paternal, and that he adored his nieces and nephews, and I saw it with my own eyes from our very first stroll around the lake that day he first met India. Of course, India is bloody easy to love, especially at that point when she was in that chubby toddler phase, but I watched him closely those first few months the three of us were together – when she had a tantrum, a meltdown, or was generally a bit naughty – and he was always calm and loving. And believe me, I was looking out for any signs he wasn't right for her, always thinking *please don't screw up, please don't say or do anything that will upset her,* and I couldn't fault him. If there was anything awry, he'd have been gone. But he only brought goodness to us.

BECOMING A FAMILY

Max and I were honest with each other from the get-go that having a kid
to think about fast-forwards all the feelings and considerations about a
new relationship a thousand times. There's no room for bullshit. There's
no faffing – it's real life. So, Max and I got pretty serious straight away,
comfortably so. When you're single without kids you can play games and
speculate, *will he call me or won't he?* I always hated that stuff, so I welcomed
this change to my dating style. It accelerated what mattered. Max is only a
few years older than me but wise beyond his years, and everything felt very
safe and steady. Before we knew it, he suggested we look for a house to buy
together, and we started living together as a family. It was really lovely. The
wholesomeness of it – making pancakes with India, scoffing popcorn on the
sofa during family movie nights. India clearly adored him as much as I did.
They say *when you know, you know*, and that's the only way I can explain the
ease with which I went from being a single mum who was scared to date to
making a family.

Max's family are incredible with India; they have been since the beginning.
I remember being very nervous about meeting them for the first time
over this big Sunday lunch along the Thames in Putney, but I needn't have
worried. He has a niece a few weeks younger than India, and the two of
them hit it off instantly. A lot of this acceptance I put down to his mum's
story. Max's older brother doesn't have the same biological dad as Max
but always has been and will be a real brother. He remembers once, when
he was young, referring to his older brother as his half-brother, and his
mum asking, 'Do you love him half as much then? That's what it sounds
like!' A question that horrified him. Of course not, he loved him as much
as his other sibling, he was just repeating an adult phrase he'd heard. That
conversation with his mum really stuck with him, it upset him. Neither of

us believe there's any reason to put a half in front of anything, or to judge different family dynamics or histories. That's the beautiful thing about modern life: you can make your families any which way that suits you and the people you choose to become a family with. There are no rules, no whispering, no judgement – well, there shouldn't be anyway.

Of course, I've had a few commenters online have a dig at me for having two different children with two different fathers. But, I mean, would these people be pleased if I stayed in a very unhappy relationship out of fear of their disapproval? I know lots of women did in the past, and some still do, but let's hope we're moving on from that. When my mum left my dad in the 1990s, because she hadn't been happy for years, she was the only one of her friends who did. Many women back then just didn't leave and will still be stuck with their husbands and no doubt will be miserable, probably having been cheated on and treated badly. What a waste of a life! Is that what you want your kids to see and normalise? Misery? Settling? Showing your children a wonderful relationship, a loving relationship, is a brilliant example for them to live by in their futures. Let's face it, happy mummy, happy everything. We mothers are the glue that holds families together. My mummy wasn't going to be made to feel guilty for bravely finding her own happiness, and neither was I. Let the *haters* judge me – I don't care. I just didn't want to be miserable. And neither should you. Make your family in a design of your choosing. Make it anything you want to be happy. Ignore the critics.

———

Showing your children a loving relationship is a brilliant example for them to live by.

———

CREATING AN LGBT+ FAMILY

LAURA-ROSE, FOUNDER OF THE LGBT MUMMIES TRIBE

The path to parenthood can be a difficult one for many, but also one filled with excitement and joy. However, trying to create your family as an LGBT+ mother or parent comes with many additional barriers, micro-aggressions, stereotypes and discrimination. If you decide to go down the adoption or fostering route, it can be a long-winded process with lots of hoops to jump through and at times you can feel interrogated. There's so many legal requirements and it can feel rather invasive, when all you're trying to do is create a family or provide a loving home for children that need it.

If you decide to have a baby of your own, either by yourself or with a partner(s), you may feel that the law and the system is not on your side or fit for purpose for people like you, from the law not supporting your path, lack of access to NHS funding, to the crippling financial burden and lack of LGBT+ competency training for professionals. And for many the barriers don't disappear once a baby arrives; we consistently have to come out as an LGBT+ family – at the school gates, the GP surgery, at gatherings, all of which can be tiresome; we are consistently 'OTHERED'.

At the LGBT Mummies Tribe, we provide a global community and support on the journey – we know all too well how difficult it can be because we have been through it ourselves over the last eleven years. Multiple failed cycles of IUI, a miscarriage, diminished fertility while managing the often daily micro-aggressions, trauma and even discrimination through our journey to motherhood – but we know how lucky we are. We have been able to birth our three miracle children between us and have the experience of both being a biological and non-biological parent, something which we appreciate many do not get the chance to do. As an organisation we are working on ensuring policies and laws are changed to create space and 'usualise' our LGBT+ families in society in a positive way, to create a more inclusive future for our children. Following organisations like ours and Stonewall will mean you are prepared for the path ahead so that you can enjoy the experience of creating your family, while knowing the barriers that you may have to overcome.

Sibling rivalry

When Wolfie came along it cemented our feelings of family – a family made from love and hard work, not blood necessarily. India and he are so sweet together, super-close – and I hope they always will be. Watching their relationship blossom is one of the sweetest joys in my life. They splash around together at bath time, he's a guest at her tea parties, a back-up dancer at her shows . . . he's her real-life dolly. And she can make him laugh like no one else.

One thing that crops up for blended siblings is the idea of favouritism. I would be very, very hot on that. Everything between both my children, regardless of DNA, has to be equal and fair. Max has assured me that he just doesn't think of the children differently. He has known India since she was eighteen months old and their bond is strong – different to his bond with Wolfie, but that is more down to their different genders than their genetics. If, as a mum, you are worried about it, I think you need to look at the trust and kindness in your relationship on a wider scale. A partner worthy of you needs to love you *and* your child. How a prospective step-parent treats your child in relation to his should be a test your partner needs to pass. Let's be realistic – 42 per cent of UK marriages now end in divorce, with children from those failed relationships entering new marriages with their parents. Blended families aren't different, there should be no shame around having half-siblings or step-parents and no one should be made to feel lesser because of your new brand of family.

Note that, personally, I don't like the term blended family; I like to think of us as one family unit rather than two coming together. But I know it's the commonly used term, so I've used it in this chapter for those who find it helpful.

BLENDED FAMILIES

GEMMA AND SOPHIA, MENTAL HEALTH, BEHAVIOUR AND WELLBEING EDUCATORS, AND FOUNDERS OF TODDLERS TEENS AND BETWEEN

To keep those special bonds within a bigger blended family, make sure you carve out special parent and child time. This can be an activity or outing chosen by the child so it becomes child-led and can either be a fixed or changed activity for that special slot each week. Try and have a value discussion about what respect looks like between half/stepchildren and step-parents and during that family discussion, discuss, compromise and then agree on these respectful values.

Building back stronger

No kid wants to see their parents go through the shit of break-ups, but in real life, it happens – and you know what . . . we probably become stronger and learn a few things because of it, as parents and children. It's how you deal with it that matters. There were positives to my parents' divorce: I wouldn't have the super-strong relationship with my mum that we have, perhaps, if we hadn't gone through that, and I wouldn't place such an importance on my mother–daughter relationship with India if I hadn't experienced that. And it's also given my mum an understanding of what I went through when I first broke up with India's father, which helped her to give me good advice and be a solid sounding board. I've got to be careful not to do some things my mother did as a single mum but the resilience I learned women have will never leave me. My advice to you is to live your life and ignore judgement. Let go of hard feelings if you can. And in all things, balance your child's happiness with your own. Just do the best you can and take the pressure off. Nothing is going to be perfect. Even if you and your partner stay together for ever, through good times and bad, that doesn't guarantee you'll have perfectly well-adjusted offspring. It's good for children to learn, in a safe way, that life does throw a storm load of shit at you that has to be dealt with. And that they can deal with it, as you can, too.

And if you have argued with a partner or ex in front of them, don't rip yourself up with guilt. I think as long as you lead with love, you can't go far wrong. They're going to hear stuff that's upsetting. They're going to see stuff that's upsetting. It's training for the horrid bullies at school, the mean bosses they'll meet at work, the bitchy mums at the school gates they'll meet when they are parents. Going through a hard time is, well, hard, but it is character building. We grow from tough times. I did. India will. We all do. The only thing we can do is love our children unconditionally and wholeheartedly.

CHAPTER FOUR

Finding Friends

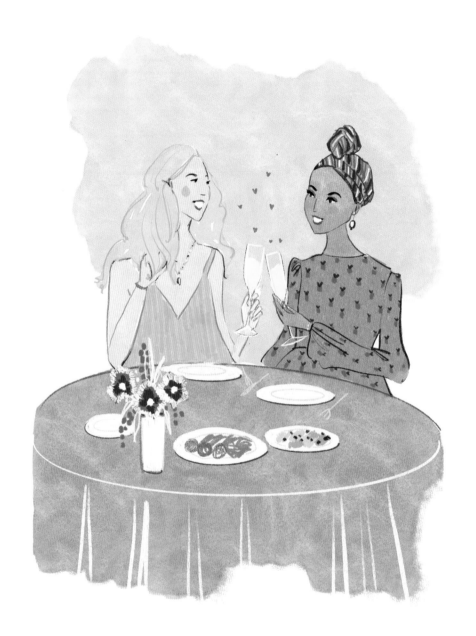

Throughout my childhood, I struggled to make friends with people at school. I had a bad learning disability, dyslexia and was always in the lowest classes, which I think, looking back, didn't help. At nursery school, I was fine! I remember being the coolest kid in the playground, all the boys wanted to hold my hand and play kiss chase with me, but at infant school, when I was a bit older, I didn't enjoy life behind the school gates at all. I was the geek with glasses and braces. I wore the cool surf brands like Quiksilver and O'Neill because my brother was a surfer dude, but just as it was starting to work, and I was starting to feel accepted, I got moved to an all-girls boarding school to finish junior school. My parents were going through a hard time, running a pub, and my mum had a lot to cope with, so thought sending me away was the best solution.

But the homesickness! I kept a chart on the wall above my bed and ticked off the days till I could see Mummy on Fridays. Don't misunderstand, it was a lovely place in Kent, a beautiful, huge, old mansion with a St Trinian's vibe, full of country bumpkins like me. We were allowed to keep horses in one of the school fields and bring pets from home (I had a rabbit called Flopsy – who I eventually sold to a friend for fifty quid to get money for the tuck shop – and a hamster called Bubbles), and five girls and I slept in a dormitory together, with trunks filled with treasures, sweets and photos from home shoved under our beds. It was lovely, very innocent with no real bullying, and it suited me down to the ground, but I was always homesick, so I left just after my parents got divorced and went to the school nearer home in Brighton that I talked about a bit in the previous chapter.

And that was hardcore. It was still a private school, but the girls there were horrible. Going from the middle of nowhere with horsey, geeky girls to a city school where the girls were all smoking, shagging, wearing full make-up, and all seemed to hate me, was a horrid time. Every morning, the girls would form a ring around me, menacingly, and I'd cry without fail, every time. Back in those days, we were all on MSN Messenger, and all the cool, popular girls would be online and I'd try to say hi and engage with them and get ignored, until one day, they replied, and said hello, and a few of them sent messages along the lines of 'We know we've been mean, and it's because you're the new girl and you're so different to us, but from this day on we're going to make an effort and we're sorry for our past behaviour.'

I was so shocked and happy, I ran to my mum and read out all these messages with a huge smile on my face. Her voice wavered as she said, 'Darling, it's the first of April. You're their April Fool.' And of course, the next day at school, nothing had changed, and a few terms later my mum removed me. Mummy used to say 'It's just jealousy, ignore them,' but obviously at fifteen, sixteen years old, you don't understand the nuances of jealousy and female behaviour, you just think there must be something wrong with you. I know why she said that – and I'll probably tell India the same if and when she experiences bullying – but at the time it didn't answer any of my questions or help really.

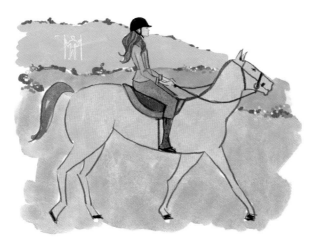

We moved back to Sussex, where I'd grown up, and I got to reconnect with my old Sussex friends, and I was finally able to create some happy memories, but bullying was still a problem. A group of teenagers decided to make posters of me and put them up around the school, a picture of chicken legs, rat-tail hair, and my face. I was always the brunt of bad things. Becoming the joker became my self-defence. My maths teacher saw what was happening and again said that word – it's 'jealousy' – but, again, I had no idea why anyone would be jealous of me.

For sixth form, Mummy somehow talked me into going to boarding school again, this time in Somerset . . . and I still find Sunday nights rank because of those memories of having to leave my family, after a lovely weekend and a roast dinner, and get on a train, on my own, to go back to school. I still hate Sunday nights because of that. I wasn't popular there either, but I got through it.

There is an upside to all this trauma: all this bullying through my childhood and teenage years, and all the counselling that I've had because of it, has actually made me such a strong person today. Now, whenever I get shit on Instagram or in the press, it doesn't affect me. So, thanks a lot, you awful bullies out there! I'll also have lots of advice to share with India and Wolfie if they ever run into this. I still don't know what I was doing wrong to be so bullied everywhere I went, but I think perhaps it was because I was a joker, and India is too, a bit of an actress. Like me, she's not going to be particularly academic, but a bit of a performer, which might make her stand out – and not always in a good way. My mama bear will kick in if it happens. Someone called her a loser at preschool last year and I wanted to track the boy down and read him the riot act. I didn't, you'll be relieved to hear.

When it comes to making friends, I suppose I'll just be open and honest with her, how I am with my mum, so she can always bring her problems to me, and she feels safe talking through her friendship dramas. You can't protect your kids from everyone and everything. And you can't be their best friend. You're their mother, not their friend. When I had these fall-outs, Mummy always told me I was right, and the other kids were always wrong, but I don't think that was a good way of dealing with it. I'll tell India to look at both sides; to put herself in other people's shoes. Tell your child honestly if they're being a bit of a dick. You won't do them any favours pretending they're perfect.

―――

You can't protect your kids from everyone and everything.

―――

Friendships made in Chelsea

I didn't go to university – a friend of my mum's had told her, 'Don't send Binky to university, it'll be like ripping up banknotes,' which was true to be fair, so I headed straight into the world of work in London at eighteen and found making friends with my colleagues easy. Me and the other receptionist would have a giggle and banter all day long, then have drinks on Friday evenings with the cool designers who worked there. Then I'd hang out with my older brother and his gorgeous friends at weekends – and got a new flatmate, Chesca Hull, who I ended up being on *Made in Chelsea* with. Then I met Ollie Locke, Gabriella Ellis and a few other people, and built a really fun friendship circle to hang out with.

It was on one of these nights out, when I was ten shots of sambuca in, that a producer pulled me to one side and said, 'We're making a show called *Chelsea Girls*, a London version of *The Only Way is Essex*, would you be interested?' Of course, I was, so we swapped details. I had a few interviews and then it was all systems go – my friends got on too – and I was suddenly in this world where my social circle was on screen, getting attention, and overnight we had fans. It got bigger and bigger, and more and more hectic, but we were young, so we were enjoying the rush of it all . . . and of course that's when the girls who had bullied me started messaging me on social media, 'Hey, how are you doing?' I ignored them, but it made me laugh. Sod you! Fake friends, no thank you. The cast of the show became my good friends; we were tight. And again, because I was bullied, and had so much counselling, I became like the onscreen therapist which made me not only popular among my colleagues but the most relatable to the public, too.

For me, going from being bullied for so many years to being a popular girl on the show – not the most beautiful, or the coolest, or the slimmest – and a favourite of the viewers was validating, and so all that bullying worked out in my favour. I'm a big believer in what is meant to be will be, and that is how I can reflect now on my struggle to find friends until I was eighteen – the pain made me a nicer person with a thicker skin, a woman who can withstand the media scrutiny and social media trolling that comes with fame. It was awful to live through, but it forced me to grow up stronger.

 # Famous friends

Some of the cast of *Made in Chelsea* were into the fame side of things, but I never was. For a start, I never know who anyone is. I'm useless at star spotting. I'd get anxiety about red carpets or being papped, it's a weird feeling, so I never sought out celebrity friends – my friends just happened to become celebrities while we were hanging out, like Rosie and Louise, and who are probably now my closest friends from the nine years I spent with *Made in Chelsea*. There was drama, there were tears, there were flings and break-ups, there was travel and parties – and it's all a bit of a blur, and weird, but I made solid friendships.

My friends on the show were shocked when a, I got pregnant and b, decided to be a mum. They didn't understand – maybe you don't until you have something growing inside you. And I get it – when your friend is suddenly on a different path to you, it can be a bit scary, and it can make you question what you're doing with your own life. I was determined it wouldn't change any of my relationships from the show, and the cast were very good and excited, but of course that wears off and once they'd done the rounds and met India, the frozen meals stopped and I felt a bit lonely. We were heading in very different directions, still fond of each other, but with different daily routines and dreams for the future.

And as you probably know, that's when you meet – and need – your new friends. Your *mum friends*. I knew one woman who had also just had a baby, who kindly introduced me to her crowd of older first-time mums, and we set up a WhatsApp group to meet for coffee, or go en masse to a soft play or park, squeeze in the occasional adult night out. These women suited my new lifestyle. I'd stopped trying to be cool, and was so happy not going out, just sitting in my pyjamas watching television. Of course, occasionally, I questioned myself and my choices: would I ever be that girl out till 3am partying again? Would I ever be the wilder Binky from the show? Maybe a bit of sadness or nostalgia snuck in on rough days, but now, despite the tiredness, I'm so happy – in myself and with the women who I call my friends.

———

You can't sit at home and expect friendships
to come to you. Get out in the world.

———

How to make mummy friends

Baby preparation classes are great. You get to talk about baby showers instead of boys and drinking, which is how I'd spent my previous decade with friends. NCT classes, or private classes, can help you find friends for life. Just make sure you look around and pick the right one. I went to a fancy one and all the women there had huge rocks on their ring finger, outrageously expensive handbags on their arm, and were all much older than me and interested in different things. I couldn't relate to any of them. It was fine, I got over it, it just pushed me to go and find friends the minute I had India.

There are apps like Bloss to help you find your tribe – go online and sign up to message boards, classes and groups – but you can find mum mates IRL too. Hang out in places where mothers and children go! Coffee shops in the morning are full of mums desperate for a decent conversation. Go to the park. There's a duck pond near where I live and I used to hang out there, waiting to see someone who looked nice to chat to. It's almost like dating. You can see a woman you like the look of, a woman with dark circles under her eyes that you recognise from your own reflection and say to her 'I feel you; I see you' – and just a brief interaction will help you feel less alone. You can't sit at home and expect friendships to come to you. Get out in the world. Admittedly, I found this hard because I was in the public eye, so I felt a bit vulnerable, but I had to be brave if I didn't want to spend those early days talking to my toaster.

Your baby can be a great prop in making friends. Baby classes can be bonding – with your baby and other parents, sharing milestones, music, story times. I was always the one scared to go somewhere on my own, eat lunch or something, but now as a mum, I am amazed by my confidence and ability to go up and talk to people. You can make friends at your child's school too – you suddenly share a language with all these other adults, and you'll never run out of things to talk about because children change so much every day. Comparing notes – supportively, not for one-upmanship – is a great connector. Now when I go out for dinner with my single friends who don't have children, I find it hard to know what to talk about. I don't want to be that parent who gets her phone out to show photos and just talks about kids' stuff, but I also just find talking to other mothers really interesting. My mummy friends and I do make an effort not to just talk about parenting. We have tequila shots and talk less about breastfeeding and more about blowjobs, making sure there's mum chat and adult chat.

Old friends are gold friends

But – and it's a big but – friends you valued before you had a baby are important to remind you who you really are, outside of the child. Try to make an effort to stay in touch. *I* need to make an effort to stay in touch. It does get harder to keep up a social life when you're a mother. For example, I've been invited out next Tuesday and I can't think of anything worse. I don't want to put my heels on, make-up on, or risk a hangover the next day . . . I'm too tired to even think about having to make adult conversation at this minute, and kids don't care if you're feeling ropy the morning after the night before. But I know I have to make the effort – that it will be good for me to dress up and go out, and that I won't regret it. Sometimes we mothers have to force ourselves not to turn into recluses.

FINDING YOUR NEW

PARTYING LEVEL

RO HUNTRISS, DIETITIAN

For some women, becoming a mother may mean that their lifestyle changes considerably, maybe from one where partying and drinking alcohol was a large part of their life. Some people may find it difficult to adjust or may at times yearn for some aspects of their old lifestyle. Just because you have become a mother doesn't mean that you can't socialise or enjoy partying or drinking some alcohol, you may just need to make a few changes to allow you to enjoy both aspects of your life. One way may be to find alternative ways to catch up with friends or socialise where you can do this without having to stay out late or drinking lots of alcohol. For example, go for a meal, arrange to go for a walk with a friend or have a games night at home. If you do go to a party, you may wish to opt for low or no alcohol alternatives, this way you can still enjoy the social aspects of the party but will wake up refreshed the next day after a good sleep ready to face the day with your parental responsibilities. If you are questioned about why you aren't drinking, have an answer ready. Remind yourself that you are doing this for you and other people's opinions don't actually matter.

Having a glass of wine in the evening can be a way to de-stress after a busy day and while this isn't a problem in moderation, if you find that the amount of alcohol that you are consuming per week is getting larger or that you are relying on alcohol to cope with stressful situations, or how much you are drinking is impacting your life in a negative way, you may want to consider reducing the amount of alcohol you consume. Tips for reducing alcohol intake:

- **Keep track of how much you drink, how often, when and what you drink –** to help you understand how you can cut down.

- **Remind yourself of why you are doing it.** Remember why you have made the decision and what your end goal is.

- **Get your partner on board** so you can both reduce your intake and get help and support from one another – it can make it so much easier.

- **There are many alcohol-free or low alcohol alternatives** on the market – find a new drink you love and don't let it stop you socialising. You can make your own mocktails or find a good white wine or spirit alternative.

- **Practise other ways of unwinding or reducing stress** – taking a bath, going for a walk with a friend, meditation, exercise classes, jigsaw puzzles, etc. Build these into your daily routine.

- **Seek support if you need it** – there are many reasons why it can be difficult to stop drinking and there are lots of ways to get support.

―――

Just because you have become a mother doesn't mean that you can't socialise or enjoy partying.

―――

How to be a good friend

Even when you're in the daily grind of motherhood, reaching out and staying in touch with people who mean a lot to you is important. It's not about grand gestures and gifts, it's about being thoughtful. Check in on them – even if just by a text or voice message, a birthday card or social post tag. Remember them. As all-consuming as your life is, other people have stuff going on too; an encouraging word from someone who loves them could make all the difference to their day. I have a friend who is suffering from really bad postnatal depression, and although I don't want to be pushy or take up her time, I want her to know I am thinking of her and that I am there for her when she does want to talk or meet someone for a walk round the park.

People who are suffering might try to push you away. I know this first-hand. I had a friend, a while ago, who was depressed after having a baby, and she was quite offish and bitchy to me. I didn't understand about postnatal depression at the time, so instead of giving her space, after some nasty comments, I thought *I'm done, sod this, you can come back to me when you're in a good mood and ready to talk to me again.* Looking back, I didn't appreciate what she was going through, and I should have stuck in there – and that experience has made me even more determined to stay connected to my friend who is currently going through so much. Just going round to say hello, sending texts, popping in to help with the baby so she can have a shower or go to the gym, help with dinner. If you're not getting through to your friend during their tough times, stay in touch with their partner or family. Just let it be known you are there for them. No matter what.

GETTING HELP FOR
POSTNATAL DEPRESSION

DR NIHARA KRAUSE, CONSULTANT CLINICAL PSYCHOLOGIST

It's important to differentiate 'baby blues' from postnatal depression (PND). Baby blues are due to hormonal dips, are experienced by 50–80 per cent of mothers and will pass. They generally start after three days from birth and last up to two weeks after the baby is born. Some symptoms include being emotional, tearful, irritable, touchy, anxious, low mood. Postnatal depression on the other hand affects around 1 in 10 women. It starts within a year of giving birth and usually within 2–8 weeks. For a diagnosis, the depression must last at least two weeks. Partners can also get PND.

These are the signs to look out for: not being able to enjoy anything, persistent feelings of sadness and low mood, hopelessness, not being able to stop crying, feelings of not being able to cope, difficulty sleeping, loss of interest in the baby, frightening thoughts – hurting self and/or hurting baby, extreme tiredness, extreme anxiety, panic attacks, loss of appetite, neglect of self-care, uncontrollable bouts of anger, lack of interest in sex. There are predictable risk factors that lead to PND so the probability of developing PND can be predicted and managed early.

What you can do:

- **Tell someone,** break the secrecy.
- **Self-care** (see the ideas outlined in Chapter Seven).
- **Take small steps to breaking the depression spiral** and every time you achieve a goal acknowledge it and reward yourself.
- **Keep a diary** – this will be a useful record to take to the doctor.
- **Access psychological help early.** Speak to your doctor.
- **Antidepressants.** Again, speak to your doctor.

I've learned the most important skill in a friend is to be a sounding board, to learn to be an effective listener. Don't talk too much about your own wonderful life if your friend is having a tough time. No one wants to hear about your perfect kid, perfect partner and your perfect world, except possibly your parents. Zip it. It's boring to gloat. That's a fact. Be mindful that other people might not feel as lucky or content as you. Especially with the reality of parenting. I'm quite good at reading people, which has become increasingly handy as I make new friends. Not everyone feels that motherhood is a blessing and the best thing that ever happened to them. Think before you speak, and don't offer advice that isn't asked for. Everyone is different so don't push your opinion to the point it sounds dictatorial or judgemental. Instead of trying to boss around a friend who isn't behaving how you would like them to, ask what they need. Distraction can be good when a friend is going through something – gossip, laugh, take them out. Be silly, be funny. It's a lovely feeling to be able to help someone who means a lot to you, and that sometimes is by doing something as simple as taking them a coffee and reminiscing about the old days.

When a friend is tired, or stressed, don't add to their unrest. Don't overstay your welcome at their house when you visit, pick up on social cues like them yawning or getting fidgety or checking their phone, and say your goodbyes. A new mum does not need you hanging around too long, expecting to be fed and watered. Before you arrive, assure them they don't need to clean up – themselves or their house – on your behalf. Wash up your own cup when you leave. Don't give them extra work to do.

Making school gate mates

I'm lucky; I feel I have my best friends now and don't really need to make any more. Even if everyone is really lovely, as the mums at India's school are! I rock up to the school gates looking like shit, and they're all glamorous. The intimidation is real. I have to remember though that everyone feels the same on the inside – even the mums who look super-confident and fabulous. We all have shit hair days and feel wretched cause we've been up all night with the kids. I've removed my judgement of them, hoping they'll do the same for me. I smile and I'm friendly, because even though I'm not searching for a new bestie, it's useful to make acquaintances with women who have kids of the same age and in the same class.

It's good to form a little gang who can help if you are running late, or don't know when World Book Day is being celebrated. I'm on a WhatsApp group with India's classmates' parents which is invaluable because I forget dates and fees, etc. We recently went for drinks after parents' evening, and I got a little bit tipsy and was worried I'd made a plonker of myself. At the school gates the next day I felt very silly, wondering what I'd said, but I think actually it was quite bonding.

———

We all have shit hair days and feel wretched cause we've been up all night with the kids.

———

There's always a couple of people you have to watch out for – that's the thing about being at your child's school – it's like being back at school yourself, with this extra element of mama bear protection. Once again, you're facing the bullies, the popular girls, and you're forced to spend time with people you have nothing in common with apart from your kids being at the same school. Don't regurgitate your past traumas from your school days. Try not to bring your emotions into their school life – don't project your shit on them. My advice to you would be avoid drama, avoid gossip, be friendly to everyone – and remember there's no rush to infiltrate groups, you'll be there with the same people for five years and you'll find your tribe eventually. If you find out you or your child hasn't been included at some after school gathering, it's natural to feel hurt, but make your own fun – instigate your own parties or outings rather than sulking and sinking into feelings from your past of being left out. I'm the only one in India's class with a blended family, so again, it makes me feel a bit intimidated, wondering what the other parents are thinking about me. But you know what I've learned? You can't know. Worrying about being judged as a mum is a whole new, huge thing – I do understand you if you're feeling nervous about groups of new acquaintances – but just keep being you, polite, friendly you . . . and worry less about what other people think.

Competitive mums

Pushy mums can grind you down. *'Oh, my little Bertie has received four Golden books from the headmaster. Has India not got one yet?'* I can spot them! I have a good radar for these women . . . and forget them! I mean, we all have it inside us to secretly think our own child is far superior to all other children. I felt it when India zoomed past the other kids at a sports school day recently – I was so proud of her I could have burst – *but* I told Max and my mum, no one else. Competitive parents are the worst, so I know who to share with, and when to shut up. These are two important skills in parenting.

My mum taught me how annoying these gloaters were. When I was little, she used to get fed up hearing about all these supermodel rocket scientist offspring of her friends, so she'd just make stuff up about me and my brother and sister. 'It's not lying, it's being more interesting with the truth,' she'd laugh it off when I questioned her. 'Jonty is doing this and that, blah blah blah,' one of her friends would drone on, and she'd respond sarcastically, 'Well, Binky's off to the Olympics tomorrow!' Total bullshit – but it shut the show-offs up and taught me never to do it. 'Darling, never, ever brag about your own children, it's the most boring thing one can ever do, and no one wants to hear it!' Of course, now she's a grandparent she wants to show off!

As long as you know how great your kids are – and more importantly, they know how great you think they are – it doesn't matter what anyone else thinks of them. Don't let other mums, or the hot air they spew about their children, deflate your confidence in your parenting skills or your child. Spend less time being competitive with other mothers, and more time competing with yourself to achieve the things that make your family the happiest and the healthiest. Know your own worth and your children's worth, irrespective of what everyone around you is doing or saying. If anything, I light-heartedly belittle India's achievements when asked. I always end up playing down what she has been up to so I can't be accused of being one of those dreadful, boasting bores. I'll say to people who ask about motherhood, 'Oh don't have kids yet – best thing in the world, but it's hard, exhausting, confusing . . .' I overcompensate the other way. There's a lot to be said about *not* showing off and being humble. You're probably raising nicer humans. And remember, there's a big difference between what you *say* and what you *do*. Let these other parents talk. They can say what they want, but it's what you actually do, and your child does, that matters.

When social media doesn't feel social

Please try not to care what people on social media say about you. I don't consider them friends, and you shouldn't either. Social media can be helpful at connecting you, informing you, and entertaining you, but don't ever think it's real. It's a curated glimpse at something people want to show you. With me, what you see is what you get, but it's hard to do that sometimes when I know some other people in my industry are faking their realness and getting likes for things that aren't perhaps fully deserved. Balancing my social media presence is a battle for me because obviously being active on it and sharing my life is my job – and how I make my money. Even when I share my real, truest self on social media, I sometimes get criticised, so I just do what is real to me, and try to ignore the disingenuous people who want to be negative about me.

Know who your friends are and don't read too much into your social media exchanges. And don't be afraid to silence or delete people. I have to be careful who I look at – if they upset me or wind me up, I mute or block them to safeguard my mental health. If I do engage with someone who has posted something nasty, I try to be nice. I've noticed the most negative people can suddenly become nice when faced with kindness – they just want attention, like most bullies you meet in person.

In general, though, I appreciate that social media mucks up your head, so only pay attention to people you value. Becoming a parent is hard enough without unleashing a whole new world of nastiness online . . . especially if they come for the kids. Max can brush nastiness off, but if I'm in self-destruct mode, I'll read some comments and regret it instantly; and if it's shit-talking about my children, I can't handle it. It's not rational to give them so much control over my mood, I know they're nasty to everyone – not discerning – looking for a reaction, but it can ruin my whole day. Honestly, these trolls . . . how do they have the time?

The ups and downs
of friendships

I don't like people not liking me. For a start, I don't think it's deserved because I'm not a bad person, and secondly negativity makes me anxious. I'm an empath, so I feel everything deeply, and I'd really be happier if everyone just got along, quieting drama and disagreements. Being an empath does have benefits – you're more compassionate, intuitive, creative, helpful – but it does mean you have to work harder to protect your heart from people who say hurtful things or end a friendship.

Being ghosted is painful. It hasn't happened to me for a long time, but your self-worth takes a battering when it does. I had lots of friend drama that really cut me up in my past, like one of my best mates shagging an ex-boyfriend of mine who she knew I still really liked. That was a double heartbreak – him and her. I'll never forget that, but I've had to forgive her to move on. When you have kids, you are more able to put the past in perspective. All those people who upset me in the past who I used to meet with anger – because I was unhappy – I don't care enough to worry about any more – because I'm happy. I've got Max and my kids, so I don't care enough to worry about them. You have to ride the waves sometimes, don't you? Everyone knows you can't be happy if you're living in the past, in pain, and that you have to move on. Wish these faux friends well and forget about them. As you get a bit older, and you become a mum, stuff like that feels more minor, and your radar for who is actually important gets stronger.

You don't give a shit about the silly things so much. Parents have bigger fish to fry. I look at these friendship tests as more life lessons and funny memories now, and I hope you can too. I honestly can't remember how devastated I was when my friend shagged my ex but at the time, I felt like my world was ending. This too shall pass. Remember that next time you're feeling bad about a friendship. As a teen, whenever I was upset by my lack of friends, or bullies saying something nasty to me, I used to tell myself, 'I won't be so upset by Tuesday; it won't hurt so badly by Sunday.' I'd tell myself there was a time frame on my upset, and it really helped in the moment and always turned out to be true. Time does heal. I guarantee you, what feels upsetting now – being excluded from a mums' night out, or your child not being invited to a birthday party – won't feel that way for ever.

In fact, with every road bump or mini drama, you learn more and more about who your real friends are, and how to value them. When someone behaves badly towards you, it'll highlight who is behaving well. There is shock and disappointment when someone who you thought you could befriend turns out to be a bit sub-par, but it can be your own version of a social experiment. That's how I'm raising India too. She's not out in full society on her own terms yet; she's friends with the children of my friends essentially. But even then, if on a playdate I suspect she's being excluded, I'll give the meanies a good telling off, then tell India to laugh at them. 'They're just silly,' I say – you can't do much more than that with a four-year-old, and I remind her to be kind, thoughtful, and to treat other people how she likes to be treated. These slightly tricky interactions are all good training for the future. I want her to be able to deal with making friends – and making enemies – in a healthier way than I did when I was young.

———

With every road bump or mini drama, you learn more and more about who your real friends are, and how to value them.

———

CHAPTER FIVE

Love
and Sex

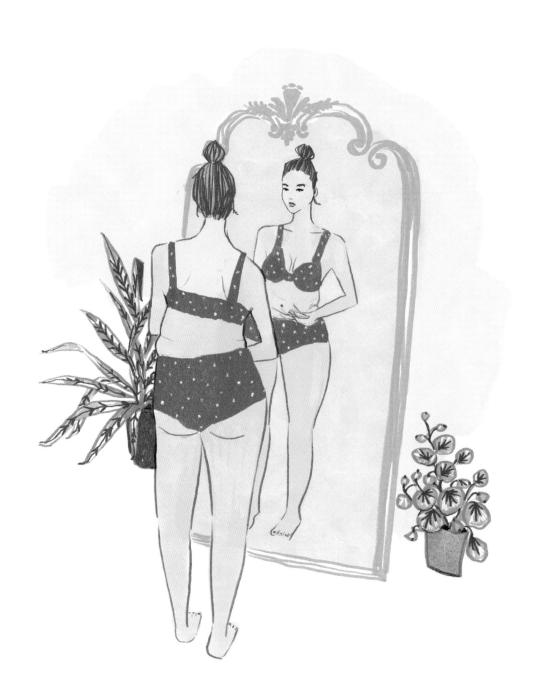

I watched a lot of Disney films when I was younger. Princes and princesses falling in love and overcoming all obstacles to live happily ever after. Truly, I'm not sure those movies did me any favours when I became an adult and had to navigate my own love life. I wish we'd followed a few of those princesses' stories past the glorious wedding day into the drudge of raising children, paying the mortgage and picking boxer shorts up off the floor. The realness might have helped brace me for the men I would later meet. I've dealt with my fair share of Prince Charming types who quickly became less chivalrous villains after the initial rush of flirting or dating. Haven't we all?

I was a little flirt at playschool and was always holding hands with someone at playtime, so sensibly, my parents kept me away from boys for as long as they could, distracting me with horses. Hormones kicked in at some point, despite their plan, and ironically my first crush was on a boy I met at Pony Club Camp. In my teen years, my best friend at the time Letty and I used to go riding together on summer days around the Sussex Downs, with a picnic bag full of snacks, and accidentally on purpose bump into boys we fancied on the beach. We'd have a snog and become obsessed and text them incessantly – but would always get freaked out if they wanted to meet again, sweating and not knowing what to do, excitedly giggling so much we'd give ourselves stitches – which isn't good when you're riding a horse – and invariably not daring to see them again. It was all silly and fun and extremely innocent.

It's taken me kissing a few frogs to appreciate not only what I do want in a relationship, but what I don't want. I've had a few relationships with some narcissistic arseholes, and I honestly don't know how I put up with them for so long. Naivety perhaps, or a misguided hope that people can change maybe? I used to think naughty boys were the sexiest boys. I was so wrong.

Now I have my 'dancing on a table' test. If you're single, think about this next time you meet a prospective partner. You're at a party and you've jumped up on the bar to dance. Do you want a partner that gets up and tries to outdance you? Do you want a partner that stands there looking at you dancing with a pleased expression on his face that says *that's my girl*? Or do you want the partner who tries to get you off the table and gives you a bollocking for being embarrassing and/or putting yourself in danger? What I've found in Max is the person who would be looking up at me with pride . . . while standing next to me in case I fell. He wouldn't be angry by my antics, he'd be amused – and concerned for my safety. The other people I've dated would be up on the table, determined to take the spotlight off me and put it on them. I've realised in my thirties that you can't have two show ponies in a relationship, and I definitely want to be the show pony. My twenties were spent with a few men who didn't like me being praised or appreciated, and that can never work long term. Your lover should adore you and be proud of you when you go out and people warm to you. Your partner should not be envious of your success and popularity, they should bask in it. I know Max does.

One of my major heartbreaks was everything I feared and more – it was horrific. And in public, played out for the world on screen in *Made in Chelsea*, me crying in bed, not knowing what to do with myself. I got cheated on a few times while I was filming and every time the producers wanted me to be told by other cast members on camera because it made good television. Even when the men I was dating weren't unfaithful they were still party boys, always out, always flirting with other women, and I couldn't handle it. Looking back, it was all age-appropriate stuff I suppose, and I got a lot out of my system and learned many valuable love lessons, like who to avoid like the plague, but it was painful to live through at the time. You do get warning bells. We have to get better at listening out for them.

When Max came along, and I could just be myself, and I could *trust* him, it felt right. Timing is everything. I was a bit too wild for him in my early twenties. I was lost, I was far too good at downing Jägerbombs, and was dealing with sudden fame, which meant I spent a lot of time talking complete crap and was mentally a bit messed up. He wouldn't have liked me back then, so I'm so glad we met when I was a mother and had got my priorities straight and had a real sense of purpose. It was easy to fall in love with each other at the point we were both at. We valued transparency and disliked games; we could be serious – not long before we met, his best friend had been killed in a freak boating accident and he openly discussed his pain – from our first date. I remember sitting there opposite him on a stool at this quiet Notting Hill bar, shaking with nerves, and not knowing what to say . . . and him just putting his hands gently on mine to reassure me that everything was okay, which I needed because I hadn't been on a date for so long and had been living on this isolated Mum Island. I didn't know if I was going to have anything to talk about with him, we had so little in common on paper, and my self-esteem was so shit at that point, but we talked, and talked, and laughed, and realised we shared the same values. He later confessed he thought it was really cute that I was so nervous.

If not a throne, then a pedestal

Max boosted my self-belief massively. He's the only man who has ever done that. From that first date, when he made me blush, talking about our future children, to today, when he still pays attention to the smallest details to make every moment extra special, I feel so lucky we found each other. He says he knew from the first moment that we would be together for ever. I finally got my Disney moments – from weekends at country hideaways to picnics in London parks, he's brought a contentment and romance to my life I once would never have dreamed of. Of course, at the beginning we had to work hard to keep things private, even though Max had been living in Hong Kong for the seven years before we met so he didn't know who I was. If anything, he finds the whole fame thing a bit cringey, so shies away from it – which is refreshing after some of the narcissistic cling-on boyfriends of my past who have loved that I was on television more than the real me. Always look for someone who can still find something to love in the messy, real, tired, grumpy you more than a projection they might have of a *fantasy* woman. You'll never be able to live up to that on a daily basis, especially in the throes of new motherhood.

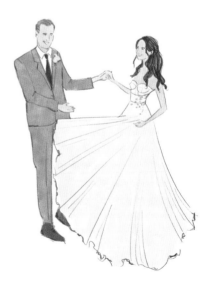

Pregnant and sexy

I know a lot of women feel super-sexy when they're expecting but I didn't during either of my pregnancies. With India, I didn't mind my bump as much because everything was new and exciting and I didn't yet realise how hard it would be to get my body back, but when I was pregnant with Wolfie, and so in love with Max, I was worried he wouldn't find me attractive any more. He never once made me feel like that – I think it was just my hormones making me unhinged. I remember being heavily pregnant and going through his iPad photos and seeing all these amazing beach parties he'd attended surrounded by these bikini-clad beauties and totally losing my shit. It was naughty of me to look but once I started, I couldn't stop, wracking my brain as to why this gorgeous guy was choosing a domestic life with a heifer like me – who came with kid and lots of random baggage – when he could be in Asia being fawned over by younger, thinner girls. I felt guilty that he'd left his single guy fun days behind him to become an almost overnight husband and father. As soon as I confessed these thoughts to him, Max laughed and called me a wally and deleted the photos, assuring me he wouldn't change his current life for anything, but I suppose once you've been cheated on and made to feel shit, the fear of it happening again never completely leaves you. And being pregnant and in love makes you all the more fragile, worried that something will spoil your lovely life when you least expect it. That isn't why we got married so quickly though. Max proposed during a beautiful countryside hike, but his reasons were practical as well as romantic. Neither of us are massively into the idea of a wedding certificate, but he thought it would be good for the kids to have that stability and that, for legal reasons, it would be the sensible thing to do. But I have found the security of being married sexy . . . and it's certainly reined in my crazy carried-away thoughts about him not being happy.

HOW YOUR BODY
MIGHT FEEL AFTER BABY

CLARE BOURNE, PELVIC HEALTH PHYSIOTHERAPIST

There are so many ways in which our body can feel different after birth, including struggles with bladder control, aches and pains in our joints, the appearance of our tummy and discomfort during sex. Research has shown that after birth 83 per cent of women report some discomfort or difficulty when returning to having sex, so if you are, you are not alone. There can be a few reasons you may be experiencing this:

• New scar tissue after a tear during vaginal delivery can be tender or tight.

• Vaginal dryness that can occur when breastfeeding due to lower levels of the hormone oestrogen.

• Granulation tissue, which is tissue that is often on top of a wound or scar, red in appearance and can feel very tender to touch. If you notice this is present after six weeks and the area is very painful, then speak to your GP.

There are also other factors that can feed into how we feel about sex after birth, including:

• Feeling less confident in our bodies.

• Not having as much time to connect with our partner.

• Feeling 'touched out' and struggling with not having much space for ourselves.

• Tiredness!

• Baby sleeping in the same room.

So, as you can see there are so many reasons that can bring barriers to us being able to relax and enjoy sex again, but if you are experiencing physical pain this is NOT normal and there IS help. Please speak to your GP or seek assessment from a pelvic health physiotherapist. They can assess your wound and vaginal tissues and give you personalised advice. In the meantime, at home, you can try:

• Using a good lubricant to help with any dryness.

• Gently massaging any new scar tissue, once it is fully healed, which is usually after six weeks but may be longer, especially if you have been treated for a wound infection. Use the technique you would have used for perineal massage before birth to gently stretch the area. It should not be painful or make the area red, but just be gentle and help to reduce tension and discomfort around the scar.

Most importantly, don't suffer in silence, reach out and get the help you deserve.

_____

Research has shown that after birth 83 per cent of women report some discomfort or difficulty when returning to having sex.

_____

Flirty thirties

Date nights are harder to come by as a mum than they are in your single and ready-to-mingle youth, so when Max and I *do* go out, I never know what to wear. At home, I wander around in holey, old jumpers and trackie bottoms, so to put on something clean, tight, *without* holes in it feels good, and I want to make an effort for him. It boosts my confidence too, to know I look good. My favourite thing to do on a night out is to dance, which makes me feel sexy. Maybe not after a thousand drinks, but a few in, I think I can carry off my moves quite well. Max doesn't dance, but he likes to watch me. We make sure the chat stays positive too. We've gone out for dinner with various friends and acquaintances where they've been so rude about each other in front of each other – and us – and it's really weird and off-putting. We try hard not to be *that* couple. Another lesson I've learned to keep my relationship with Max healthy is to never go to sleep on an argument. I'm stubborn but I hate lying in bed next to him and not speaking, it's the worst feeling ever and I just can't do it any more. It feels really lonely. Life is too short; our relationship is too valuable.

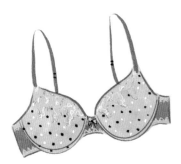

SEXUAL CONNECTIONS

KATE MOYLE, SEXUAL AND RELATIONSHIP
PSYCHOTHERAPIST, PSYCHOSEXOLOGIST AND HOST
OF THE SEXUAL WELLNESS SESSIONS PODCAST

A huge challenge for parents is finding the time to feel like a couple again. The work of parenting is never done, and often while babies and children take an obviously huge amount of time and attention, it's the invisible workload that is paired with parenting which is also a drain on our energy and time. Like every other area of our lives, our sex lives and relationships need attention and nurture, it's not a Disney movie where they 'just happen' and some of the hardest, but most rewarding work that we can do in our lives is in our intimate relationships. For many reasons we don't see that represented around us, and this can mean that when we are struggling in our relationships that it feels like it's just us, or when conversation feels like it's only about the children, or the to-do list, we can yearn in some way for the us that we used to be. There is a term – matrescence – which we use to describe the transition to motherhood, socially, physically, emotionally and hormonally, and to understand that we go through a transition both individually and in our relationships; we therefore shouldn't expect our relationship not to change too.

So when thinking about making time to connect and invest in our relationships, the first step is that we have to make it happen. Like anything in our lives, it won't just magically appear or turn up, we have to go to it. We book in meetings at work, organise holidays, make time to see friends, and arrange baby classes – our relationships need the same investments. The first step is to make time. It sounds simple and many people push back on the idea of booking in or scheduling couple time but try to reframe it from scheduling to prioritising. Make the time, put the screens and distractions away, and focus on each other. Non-verbal forms of communication such as eye contact and touch are powerful ways of building connection and eye contact has even been used by researchers to trigger feelings of love.

We also talk about taking appropriately named baby steps back into sexual experiences to re-establish sexual and intimate contact. Many mothers can experience what's called touch fatigue where they feel 'touched out', and sex can feel like a part of that. Try and make time to just lie or sit together on a bed or a sofa and talk, touch and kiss without any expectation of it going anywhere. The intention is to build little connection bridges between you, without the pressure of it having to become sexual or lead to sex. These experiences can help to trigger responsive desire, which is a real boost for your sexual wellbeing. Opening up your definitions of sex can be really helpful here too, focusing on what feels good, as particularly in the postnatal window you may not be feeling ready or up for intercourse. Sexual experiences come in all different shapes and sizes and finding what works for you and following what feels good has emotional, psychological and physiological rewards.

———

*Non-verbal forms of communication
such as eye contact and touch are
powerful ways of building connection.*

———

Dating your partner

It's hard to stay connected when you have young children – and I don't love traditional dates at the best of times. They feel quite false when you already live with your partner, sitting in an intense environment, staring at someone you're with all the time anyway. But I appreciate it's a nice thing to do – and an important thing to do when our lives are getting busier and busier, and romantic connections can go haywire. I think the main thing for Max and me isn't the setting, but the ability to talk to each other, so our favourite type of date is going for a long dog walk, out in the fresh air, zero pressure, no one interrupting us. We love weekends away in the countryside, drinking wine in front of a log fire, and we even like putting the kids to bed and getting cosy at home, him cooking while I chat away drinking champagne. We just really enjoy each other's company. It's like we're best mates, which I guess we should be. That's the dream, right? My point is that date nights don't have to be flowers and fancy restaurant reservations, you don't have to be in full face make-up and high heels. You just have to be focused on each other, which gets harder and harder in the distracted world of parenting.

Work it, baby

There are ups and downs in all relationships, and you really have to focus on being kind and affectionate to each other, even when you're in the weeds of new parenthood, making sure the reasons you fell in love aren't forgotten and your love doesn't wilt. When times are tough, you've got to try and remember you're on the same side; you're each other's cheerleaders. Max is my biggest motivator. He gets me excited about new opportunities, gives me ideas about work projects, thinks about connections I should make. I've never had more respect for a man in my life, I'm really proud to be married to him . . . and I hang on to that fundamental truth even when we're tired and squabbling about the washing-up or some little niggle I know I won't even remember the next day.

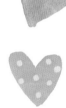

I feel like I'm in my first grown-up relationship, where both people are equally invested in long-term goals. I've never had this before, which is probably why I was so scared at first. I didn't want to lose him! But I knew enough about him to know he wanted the real Binky; he didn't want a performing, fake Stepford Wife type. I know when some women are scared of losing their men they act in a certain way, dress in a certain way – forget about what they need in a bid to appear perfect for their man and what he needs. I know women like that, who have got big breast implants because their man wants them or wake up an hour before him to apply a full face of make-up and blow-dry their hair. Exhausting, right? If you want some new boobs or a perfectly made-up face, then go for it – I just don't have the energy! Of course, we all do that a bit on the first few dates, putting our best side forward, but in a marriage? I could not be a trophy wife – I'm too lazy. It can work for some – she gets plastic surgery for him, he gets a closet full of designer handbags for her – and good for you if you find each other; but don't become someone's puppet, and don't do all the showy stuff to post a fake life on social media. When women have to post constantly about how amazing and generous their husband is, my suspicious mind goes into overdrive. What are they hiding or overcompensating for? I'm happy with Max treating us to experiences, like family weekends away, and the occasional bunch of flowers.

But the sexiest thing we can give each other is our ears: listening. We listen out for what the other one is saying and what they're *not* saying. I'd hate to get divorced. The idea really scares me. I know it feels like 99 per cent of all couples get divorced eventually, especially if they don't put the work in, and I don't want to be part of that statistic. Friends who have put the work in, and go to couples therapy, never regret it. They say it's good to put the work in before everything breaks down beyond repair. Don't be ashamed to admit you need help; or you need someone external to the emotions within the relationship to dissect what should change. I'd be up for it if our communication became difficult. I'd never say never. Going to therapy doesn't mean you've failed – quite the opposite. It means you're tired, you're stressed, you're stuck, you're juggling a hundred different balls in the air . . . but you want to save what you have. You want new ideas. You want to get out of the rut you're in. New communication, old partner.

And I say all this with the added caveat that sometimes couples therapy doesn't work – but that can be good too. Sometimes people are just ill-suited, or grow in different directions, and would both be happier out of the binds of that particular relationship. It can make you understand why it's not working, and so rather than keep banging your head against a wall, you have the tools and the strength to end things and move on in a healthier way. Better to find that out sooner rather than later. This happened with India's father. We had therapy, and it made us both appreciate our relationship was never going to work, and we moved on, focusing on India's wellbeing.

THE HARDEST
PARENTING DECISION:
SLEEP OR SEX?

LETO, PELVIC HEALTH PHYSIOTHERAPISTS,
PRE- AND POSTNATAL EXERCISE SPECIALISTS
AND WOMEN'S HEALTH EXPERTS

THE MEN SAY THEY'RE TIRED BUT YOU'RE THE ONE UP MOST OF THE NIGHT. You spend hours pumping milk and they chuck it away without thinking. You think they're living it up at work all day, they think you're lounging around on the sofa. When your limitless and free-range life has been replaced with the routine tasks and responsibilities that come with parenthood, your spontaneous desire is understandably reduced. But that's okay! Even if you're not ready for sex, you can work on connection. Don't worry about what other couples are doing and think instead about what's right for you.

COMMUNICATION WITH YOUR PARTNER IS KEY. Share your fears and anxiety around your recovery and have a realistic conversation on how it might impact your intimate life. When you do feel ready, it might help to remember that sex is much more than vaginal sex. 'Sex' can be holding hands and kissing passionately, or intimately touching each other for a few minutes.

WORK ON YOUR SLEEP RATHER THAN SEX FIRST. Being deprived of sleep can trigger hormonal changes which make your libido go AWOL. If you're breastfeeding, you'll also be producing a hormone called prolactin which helps milk production but can dampen desire. Accept any offers of help from trusted people to help you rest and recover, night or day! Delegate some night feeds to your partner. If you're breastfeeding exclusively, ask if they can handle the night-time nappy change and winding to give you some extra sleep. And crucially, don't try to do much. Do you really need to take three buses across town with your buggy to go to an event you don't even really want to go to?

MIX IT UP. At the right time, post-birth intimacy can also be an opportunity to mix it up while your body recovers. You could try gentle foreplay, clitoral stimulation and 'outercourse' rather than intercourse. Use a lubricant to make it all a lot smoother and more fun. Sex should not be painful. Life is too short to put up with pain. If you are experiencing pain with sex, a specialist pelvic health physiotherapist can help. They can conduct an internal vaginal examination to assess the type of trauma your muscles have gone through, and tailor your treatments accordingly. This might include gentle manual therapy to release tension on the scar tissue or surrounding areas, manual sensory work, biofeedback, and breathwork which can really help with returning to sex. And remember with intimacy, it's the little things that count. Do you have any time to hang out together and have fun? This is important even in the early days. Could you do something together like a new walking route, or a short, gentle yoga session at home? Offer a massage and get one in return, it might lead to a sleep, or some sex, either way it's a step in the right direction.

_____

Don't worry about what other couples are doing and think instead about what's right for you.

_____

Passion play

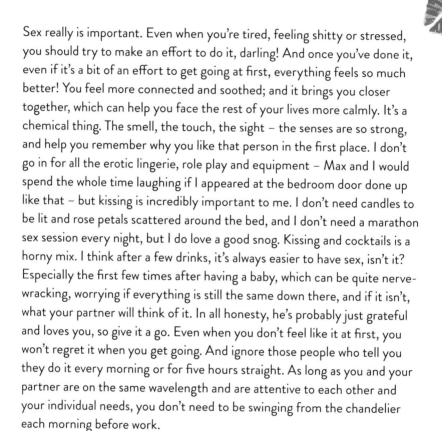

Sex really is important. Even when you're tired, feeling shitty or stressed, you should try to make an effort to do it, darling! And once you've done it, even if it's a bit of an effort to get going at first, everything feels so much better! You feel more connected and soothed; and it brings you closer together, which can help you face the rest of your lives more calmly. It's a chemical thing. The smell, the touch, the sight – the senses are so strong, and help you remember why you like that person in the first place. I don't go in for all the erotic lingerie, role play and equipment – Max and I would spend the whole time laughing if I appeared at the bedroom door done up like that – but kissing is incredibly important to me. I don't need candles to be lit and rose petals scattered around the bed, and I don't need a marathon sex session every night, but I do love a good snog. Kissing and cocktails is a horny mix. I think after a few drinks, it's always easier to have sex, isn't it? Especially the first few times after having a baby, which can be quite nerve-wracking, worrying if everything is still the same down there, and if it isn't, what your partner will think of it. In all honesty, he's probably just grateful and loves you, so give it a go. Even when you don't feel like it at first, you won't regret it when you get going. And ignore those people who tell you they do it every morning or for five hours straight. As long as you and your partner are on the same wavelength and are attentive to each other and your individual needs, you don't need to be swinging from the chandelier each morning before work.

Quality is more important than quantity for most of us in the bedroom, which is just as well because being a parent does tame things down a bit. India will want to creep into the bedroom occasionally and snuggle down in the middle of the bed; Wolfie will be up yelping in the small hours because he's teething. Your sex life is going to change. Just try and remember every now and again to connect as adults – not just parents. And if you need help, get it. My friend down the road never wanted to shag her husband until she started watching erotic television shows with hot Australian actors in it. Now they're back better than ever, non-stop. Her husband can't believe his luck after such a long dry spell. So, if watching or reading erotica, or buying yourself sexy lingerie, or sending a cheeky WhatsApp while you're at work, or hiring a babysitter and going for a meal, or begging your in-laws to have the kids for the night so you can stay in a hotel makes you feel saucier – do it. Do it before you forget how lovely it can be to be intimate with someone you love. Oh, and the biggest turn-on? Talking to each other nicely. You can't expect to bicker and grumble and put someone down all day then to get it on in the evening. Try and talk to your partner how you would like to be spoken to. Respect is the biggest aphrodisiac.

Men and libido

There's an outdated notion still hanging around that men are always up for sex, and it's the women who cry headache. In my friendship group, this is not the case – anything from work stress to taking protein shakes at the gym to necking hair loss pills can depress a man's libido and testosterone. Why would we expect men to have a constant erection when they have a lot on their plate – making a living, raising a family, looking after ageing parents? An issue is that while women tend to talk to their friends and read books, blogs or magazines about relationships, men internalise a lot of anxiety . . . which further depletes their libido. New dads might also be feeling a bit left out. They're your number one guy one minute, then baby

– or babies – arrive and they quickly drop to the bottom of your priority list. They can feel a bit jealous, and their fall in stature may even affect their self-confidence. A relationship counsellor friend told me that the cheaters aren't the super-libidinous guys, but the ones who are most insecure and cheat to feel wanted and sexy again. They need validation outside of their marriage. Clearly, this does not solve anything, but it made me think again about how important it is to stay connected.

The sexier second act

This too shall pass. The constant exhaustion, the children crawling into your bed every night, the worrying about doing your Kegels . . . you'll have a whole second act when the kids have grown up. You can go back to being a bit wilder, spontaneous and romantic then, so make sure you maintain intimacy, even if it's once a fortnight with the lights out. Parenting is just your first act. Don't be hard on yourself, or your partner. Try and remember in those moments when you bitch and snap that it's probably because you're tired and you haven't slept, and don't be afraid to reach out with an apology and a hug. Once the connection is gone entirely, it's hard to get it back. You can forget how good it feels to hold hands, kiss, get naked. Yes, you're a mum . . . but before you know it, they'll be gone, and you and your partner will be left alone together. Max and I are actually excited for this. Because we met when I'd already had India, we never had that wilder, freer, honeymoon phase that other people have. We talk about our second act on our occasional date nights – where we'll travel, what we'll see. Remember you are not just parents, you're partners.

ANSWERS TO THE MOST
FREQUENT POST-BABY
SEX QUESTIONS

CLARE FAULKNER, SEX AND RELATIONSHIP THERAPIST

1. Is it true our vaginas will feel different during sex after baby?

It's important to remember that we are all different and our own unique experience is just that, unique! Yes, it is true that some women may report a difference but not every woman will. A change may be expressed as a difference in sensation (heightened or less sensitive), the vagina may feel loose or wider, lubrication may have changed, or soreness might be present. The difference may reflect what happened during the birth, for example, a perineal tear or damage to the pelvic floor.

2. Is it true that most women are likely to experience discomfort during sex after having a baby?

No, on the whole I would say this isn't true. It's important to give the body time to heal. Usually once the GP signs you off at the six-week appointment much of the necessary healing has taken place. However, try not to feel pressure and rush it. If it hurts it won't be enjoyable, which slightly defeats the object! It's totally normal not to be wanting sex straight away – you have a tiny new human to look after who is probably keeping you up all night! If pain does persist it might be worth discussing it with your GP who can check that everything is healing as it should.

3. What about if you had a C-section, are you still likely to experience discomfort?

Just because you had a C-section doesn't mean the pelvic floor has got away unscathed. Regardless of the type of birth, I still recommend pelvic floor exercises (also called Kegel exercises) after birth for women. Pelvic floor exercises help to tone the vaginal muscles as well as the pelvic floor. Specialist woman's health physiotherapists can do internal examinations to check the damage and recommend exercise programmes post-birth. Speaking from personal experience, I found this to be very useful. My physio carried out ultrasound imaging of the pelvic floor muscles as well as a perineal evaluation. No woman wants a future prolapse, so I would advise investing shortly after delivery.

4. Is it true we don't need birth control if we are breastfeeding?

This is a myth. Breastfeeding should not be used as a method of birth control as it's not a reliable option. Neither should you rely on waiting until you get your period back. Pregnancy can occur as soon as three weeks after birth, so please speak to your GP or practice nurse about contraception.

5. Is it true that it is likely to be quite dry down there?

It is normal to experience dryness after birth. This is due to the reduced levels of oestrogen compared to pregnancy. Breastfeeding further depletes levels, so this is worth considering when assessing your vaginal dryness. Women should find that once periods return, oestrogen levels increase, which should help any issues. Dryness has a tendency to increase with age, so a natural change in your body might be inevitable. If this is the case, you can use lubricant. I recommend YES, the organic intimacy company. They do a range of organic lubricants including water-based or plant-oil-based options. Do note that oil-based lubricants may not be suitable with condoms, so please check before use. Their vaginal moisturising gel can also be used daily to hydrate and relieve vaginal dryness and discomfort.

6. Can orgasms actually be better after a baby?

Some women do report that birthing awakens their genital area, and they report more sensitivity. Some couples may experience a new intimacy as a result of becoming parents, which has a positive shift on the relational space. This then feeds their sex lives. Professionally I would say that most couples experience a new baby as a passion killer, so please don't doubt yourself if you are not feeling ready for sex.

7. I've heard that some women simply cannot stand to be touched after having a baby – is this true?

Yes, and this is something I have experienced in my practice. There are many reasons and factors to consider with this. For example, birth trauma, relationship issues, a psychosexual presentation, postnatal depression, and exhaustion to name but a few. Not wanting to be touched in the initial months is quite normal, but if this persists, consider discussing it with a professional as well as your partner.

8. Is it normal to feel totally unsexy after having a baby?

Absolutely. For some women, their new curves look and feel very different to their pre-baby body. There are the changes to the vagina, which we have touched on, plus aching boobs which may tend to leak when you don't have your (unsexy) feeding bra on. Then there is the psychological element. New mums have a new identity and role to integrate while attempting to hold on to their individualism. The relationship narrative might be one of snappiness, irritability, sleep deprivation and lack of time and space, all of which leaves less desire for intimacy. On the whole babies don't tend to be passion makers, so if you are having sex at all you are doing well! It will come back, eventually, but for now it's totally normal to be focusing on your new bundle of joy.

CHAPTER SIX

Body Confidence, Diet and Exercise

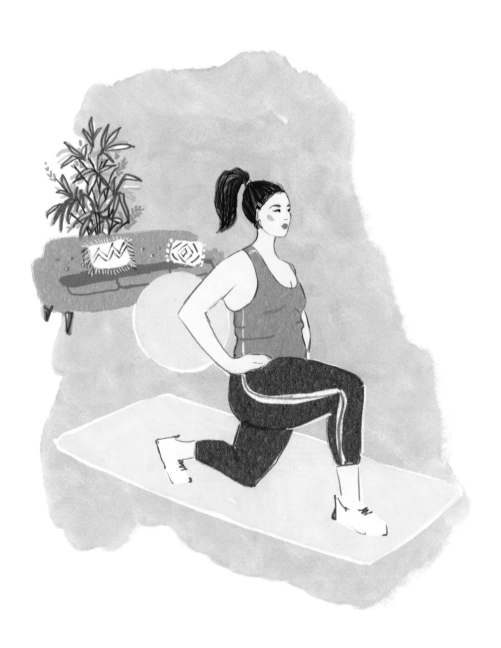

When I was a teenager, I started to notice my hips were a little wider than other girls my age, but I really loved food and knew losing weight would mean restricting myself, so I wasn't compelled to do anything about it. I was an active child and teenager, having horses and an outdoorsy life, and it was bred into me to value good health rather than a skinny appearance. Of course, moving to London changed my outlook on many things and a bit of self-doubt about my body crept in. I was starting to drink more and was getting a little heavier – and it didn't help that I was hanging around more with my big brother who always seemed to be surrounded by supermodel, gazelle types. He bought me a gym membership, which was his not-so-subtle way of telling me I was getting a bit porky … but still, I was enjoying myself too much to actually care enough to change my habits. And when I joined *Made in Chelsea*, the partying and drinking went up another notch.

Still, my parents always had crisps and chocolates dotted around the house and eating them was never a big deal. Instead of viewing certain foods as treats or rewards, or being fascinated with food, my mother's mantra of 'everything in moderation' became the rule I would follow, and still try to follow – and instil in my children – to this day.

BODY TALK

GEMMA AND SOPHIA, MENTAL HEALTH EDUCATORS
AND FOUNDERS OF TODDLERS TEENS AND BETWEEN

When you discuss your body, remember that
your children will hear and then internalise what
you're saying about yourself and may begin to
feel that way about themselves! Use adjectives
like strong, powerful, soft and fleshy as examples
of parts of your body – positive and accurate
descriptions your little ones will hear and then
believe about your body and theirs. Reframe
discussion about exercise to be about keeping
strong, or flexible or dedicated or joyful, so it is
seen as a pleasure and a way to maintain positive
mental health rather than to burn off food or
achieve a certain look.

Falling in love with fitness

A great advantage of becoming a reality television personality is the jobs and opportunities that come your way. One of my first bits of work was with a protein company, who introduced me to a personal trainer, who I really hit it off with. I started drinking their shakes because I wanted to, not just because I got paid to drink them, and I started spending time around people who kept talking about this thing called a 'fitness bug' – they said once you had it, you'd never lose it, but I didn't have a clue what people were talking about for the first few years of socialising and partying, filming and travelling . . . And then it happened. I caught the bug.

I remember filming in Cannes in the south of France for two months with the rest of the cast the summer before I had India. Josh and I had just split up, but despite being in a mentally tough place, I'd just got the biggest job ever: being the Reebok UK women's ambassador, which I took very seriously. While my castmates spent their mornings lounging around the villa eating croissants and drinking mimosas, I jumped on this shitty little exercise bike in the villa's hot, sweaty garage and pedalled hell for leather for hours. And I loved how it made me feel, and I loved how it made me look. That's when I truly realised how exercise – and the endorphins it releases – is just as much for the mind as the body. I felt like I could handle anything life threw at me, which was just as well, because it was about to throw something massive in my direction: an unexpected, unplanned pregnancy.

I spent months training hard for the Reebok campaign, but on the day I headed into the studio to do the photoshoot, I was disappointed to see that I had a little pot belly. I was nine weeks pregnant with India, not that I knew that at the time. Reebok weren't exactly over the moon when I did discover

I was pregnant and told them, but we agreed to do a post-baby shoot eleven weeks after I'd given birth, which, as you can probably imagine, I thought would be a great incentive to lose the baby weight and get in shape.

Oh, how naive I was to think this would be easy! Eleven weeks is no time to get back in shape – specially to head up a massive global brand fitness shoot! You're not even sleeping properly at that point. But I'd made a commitment to them and myself, and after getting physiotherapists to check me out internally – I had a small prolapse with Wolfie but was okay after India – and externally to make sure I could work out again, I went for it. I looked terrible. I felt I did, anyway. And when I got the all clear to do jumping jacks and burpees again, I got back into it.

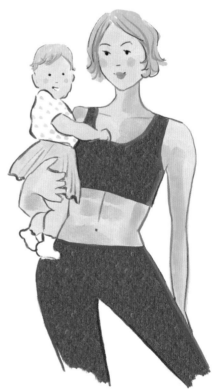

EXERCISING AFTER BABY

CLARE BOURNE, PELVIC HEALTH PHYSIOTHERAPIST

Returning to exercise and feeling stronger again after pregnancy and birth is so important for so many reasons, but it is essential that we do it the right way. The six-week time frame that we often hear we need to wait before we return to exercise is not a magic timeline, but purely the average time for soft tissue healing. It is important that we allow our bodies time to strengthen and rehabilitate as part of our return to fitness journey. A key part of this is our pelvic floor strength, and sometimes if we return to certain exercise too soon, especially impact exercise, we can experience symptoms of incontinence or prolapse. So here are a few top tips on how to get back into exercise happily and without symptoms:

- Ensure you are working on pelvic floor exercises daily. Start sitting and lying but build up into standing.

- Start with low impact exercise, for example, bodyweight movements such as squats and lunges, cycling and swimming, postnatal Pilates or yoga.

- Latest guidelines suggest that the earliest we should be returning to running is twelve weeks postpartum, as long as we have done pelvic floor rehabilitation and have no symptoms. For many it is likely to be after twelve weeks before they are ready to run.

- You can exercise when breastfeeding, just make sure you have a good supportive sports bra, keep well hydrated and make sure you are supporting yourself with the right nutrition.

- Starting slow and building up is the best approach, but it can feel frustrating at the time. If you experience any pain, incontinence of your bladder or bowels, a heaviness or dragging sensation in the vagina, a bulging up or dropping down of the tissues down the middle of your tummy, then please don't push through. Seek assessment by speaking to your GP or finding a pelvic health physiotherapist privately and know that there is help for all of these symptoms.

The brain boost

Those first few months with India are a massive blur. I found a post I'd shared on Instagram recently, just after India was born, and it was something like, *you may be feeling lonely right now and that all you are is a mother, but remember you are everything to your baby.* I must have needed to tell myself that; I must have been feeling quite discombobulated. Many of us feel like we're not ourselves any more, just a machine who puts all their focus on a child and loses their identity. We're tired and overwhelmed with love and fear . . . and anything you can do to help your mental health is powerful.

One thing I'd say to new mums who are struggling to get motivated to exercise – not everyone has the threat of public humiliation via photoshoot to get them to toe the line and get in shape – is to understand the mental benefits. Getting to the gym or going for a run is a good way to be on your own, away from the responsibilities of motherhood, and have some me-time focused on yourself and not everyone else who normally demands your attention. When I had India, I found a gym down the road from where I was living called the Harbour Club, and it had a crèche. I'd put her in there and do a 45-minute session and feel so much better for it, top to toe. You have to use every tool you can find during those first few months to feel good about yourself.

I didn't feel extra pressure to lose the baby weight because I was in the public eye, even though I was the first one of our *Made in Chelsea* group to get pregnant but I remember, that summer I had India, all my female castmates wearing tiny crop tops and little summer dresses and feeling rank and lumpy standing next to them. I thought I looked awful, but with hindsight I know I didn't look awful at all, I looked like I'd just had a baby!

But my identity was completely gone. I couldn't really compare my body or myself to anyone in the same age bracket because I was the first one in my gang to have a baby, and I was a bit anxious about when I'd get back to my old self, in my old clothes. But I did the most important thing a new mum can do, I didn't rush. I did some pelvic floor exercises. I never used to wee when I ran but obviously that is a big thing for many women post-pregnancy, so Kegels are a necessary evil.

It was probably around India's first birthday that I finally felt back to my old self, fit and strong. I'd started doing F45 training, these high intensity group workouts that were fast and fun and really changed my body – so much I got a *Woman's Health* magazine cover, which was another incentive to shape up further. I was smashing it! I'd wake up, have a black coffee, drop India at nursery – which was a massive help to my mindset, oh my God! – and then head to F45. I wasn't eating carbs; I wasn't eating sugar, which with hindsight might have been a bit too obsessive! People started to say I was getting a bit too thin, but I didn't think so at the time. Looking back, I think I may have dabbled with body dysmorphia after having India; I think I still do slightly perhaps. But I am aware of how my brain can make me think a certain way about how I look which isn't based in reality. I check in with myself to stop going down slippery slopes of self-loathing, or being too hard on myself, or caring too much about what is going on externally, rather than internally. We all need to look at ourselves kindly. Women are often their own harshest self-critics, which is very sad.

BODY IMAGE AND POSITIVITY

EMILY ANDREW, MOVEMENT AND MENTAL HEALTH
PRACTITIONER AND CERTIFIED COACH

Body acceptance is something that really helped me to stay curious about the way that pregnancy affected my weight and shape, instead of panicking, being self-critical and falling into the comparison trap. The urge to try to 'bounce back' can be overwhelming but it's important to remember that your body is entirely individual, incredible and deserves love, praise and compassion. Get informed so you can understand the changes happening to your body and don't feel totally lost and can instead move through without judgement. Reframe negative thoughts. It's natural to have days where you're just not feeling it but instead of beating yourself up and telling yourself you're failing, allow yourself to feel it. Then, as you would with a friend, try to reframe the negative into a neutral or positive thought. You could practise gratitude and every day write down three good things that you're grateful for – even better if they relate to your body. This helps to build a more positive narrative and strengthen your resolve on those days when it's a struggle.

Move your body in a way that you enjoy and makes you feel good, not based on how many calories it burns or because the latest influencer told you to, and surround yourself with people who lift you up and make you feel good. If you are constantly listening to negative comments from others, it can be a total drain mentally and really start to affect your body image. Bring those who encourage and support you close and let others fall away. And give yourself a break. Be gentle with yourself – kindness and self-compassion are key. Remember you are doing a great job. When I realised that my baby was going to benefit from the years of work that I had put into myself, that they would be able to talk to me about anything and I would be able to understand and support them no matter what, I knew that I could handle whatever my pregnancy could throw at me.

Lastly, if you've experienced poor mental health in the past, it's common to feel worried about pregnancy and the postnatal period. Postnatal depression is thankfully widely spoken about, helping to break unhelpful stigma, however, pregnancy after living with an eating disorder or disordered eating is still very hush hush, despite many women experiencing one or the other at some period in their lives. After living with bulimia, anorexia, depression and anxiety in my early twenties and being recovered for over seven years, I found myself contending with stressful thoughts and feelings as I had severe morning sickness for most of my pregnancy. The fear that you are relapsing, the concern that you are going to hurt or lose your baby and the worry that you aren't eating enough or eating too much can be paralysing. The most important thing is to talk to someone, whether it be your partner or a professional. Eating disorders and mental illnesses thrive in secrecy, so the sooner you talk about how you feel, the better. Reach out for help, get in touch with your midwife or GP and ask them to get you in touch with your perinatal mental health team who are available until your baby is one. Nourish yourself – if you need to revert to a meal plan, eat little and often or invest in a nutritionist, find a way that you can nurture yourself and your baby.

---

*It's natural to have days where
you're just not feeling it.*

Team up

I met Max in the January, and the issue of *Woman's Health* with me on the cover looking really fit came out in the February. I thought I looked so good when I met him, but he says I was too skinny when we first met – and I remember at the time thinking that I still needed to lose more weight. When I got pregnant with Wolfie, I wasn't worried because I knew what to expect and I was in a better place mentally, supported by Max – and I didn't eat as badly during that pregnancy. With India, I didn't know what would be happening to my body, and how hard it would be to get it back. I was like, 'Right, this is the one time I can eat anything and everything,' and really went for the whole *eating for two* thing, which is bollocks. Whereas, with Wolfie, I knew to enjoy it but not go too mad. I carried on working out through my pregnancy with him, which I was too scared to do with India. If you're fit before, of course you can continue to train when you're pregnant, but I didn't realise that! My cravings were different too. With India it was everything sweet – and believe me, I went to town! With Wolfie, it was everything beige, with added Marmite and pickled onion crisps, but I knew not to stuff myself quite so much. Once I had him, I'd go for nice lunches, but started eating better and training again much sooner than I had with India. Second time round, I understood what I could and should do much better.

———

You get the endorphin rush and the knowledge you are doing something to push you in the right direction.

———

148

Getting back in the gym

It can be intimidating going to the gym for the first time after having a baby, and being surrounded by beautiful people, bright lights and big mirrors. I remember looking at my reflection on the first day back after Wolfie's birth and thinking, 'Bloody hell, I've got a long way to go!' A bit scared off, I did a few workouts in my garden, where I could look rank and no one but my poor trainer would have to look at me. Max and I got married seven weeks after I'd given birth to Wolfie and we went on a little last-minute babymoon to Spain afterwards because we had the post-wedding blues, and I distinctly remember thinking I looked all right in my bikini, but looking back I didn't. Not really. And that is fine and to be expected . . . I'd just grown a human in me! I recorded my early garden workouts and popped them up on Instagram to share and to help motivate my followers, and to show them that your body doesn't bounce back straight away, that it does take effort, and that's fine. Don't hate on yourself. Still, I don't enjoy being bigger and I was determined to get rid of my baby weight. I actually shocked myself how much my self-confidence was affected by my appearance. When I was pregnant, I thought the worst all the time, to the point Max thought I was psychotic because I was so full of self-loathing. I thought he'd run off with someone skinnier than me. I felt revolting and that he could go and find another girl and have a lovely life with her because I was just fat. And that was crazy. I'd lost all grip on reality. And again, that's where exercise helps – it makes you mentally and physically stronger and able to cope with your new life as a mum, and if you're working out, even if you're not seeing immediate results, you get the endorphin rush and the knowledge you are doing something to push you in the right direction.

YOUR OPTIMUM TIMELINE

FOR POSTNATAL FITNESS

REHABILITATION

ZOE ROBSON, PILATES INSTRUCTOR AND
FOUNDER OF FIT MUMS BERKSHIRE

PELVIC FLOOR REHAB: Whether you had a vaginal or C-section delivery, your pelvic floor went through a lot supporting the added weight of your bump during pregnancy. For vaginal deliveries you may also have stitches. Performing Kegels can actually help aid recovery due to increasing blood flow to the area. Ideally start doing Kegels one week after delivery. Practise three times a day, performing 10 x squeeze and releases and 10 x 10-second squeeze and holds.

RECONNECTING TO YOUR CORE: Learning to connect your breath with core engagement is your secret weapon to help get your core muscles strong again. Inhale, relaxing your pelvic floor and tummy muscles and then as you exhale, draw your pelvic floor and belly button in and up. Repeat for 15 breaths and perform this twice a day. This type of core connection breathwork can be done straight away after vaginal delivery. For C-section mamas, I would advise giving your scar a couple of weeks to heal first so you aren't putting any pressure on your stitches.

WALKING: A great exercise as it's low impact and gets you outside. Walks can start whenever it feels comfortable for you. Start with a slow pace and short distances. If you feel any pain or discomfort, it's a sign you might need to take a break or stop. Gradually build up both the distance and speed over time.

POSTNATAL CLASSES AND BODYWEIGHT EXERCISES: Around six weeks postnatal onwards you may wish to return to classes or the gym. Pilates and yoga are good options as both are slower paced and focus on working with the breath. It's best to find a specific postnatal class or trainer. Bodyweight exercises such as squats and lunges are normally fine to start at the 4–6-week mark.

ADDING WEIGHTS: If you like to use weights, these should only be used after you have had clearance from your doctor to return to exercise. Also, you should have worked through the rehabilitation stages above to ensure you have a solid foundation of pelvic floor and core strength first. If adding resistance, start with light weights, low reps and take adequate rests between sets so you can build up safely and gradually.

HIGH IMPACT EXERCISE: Pursuits like running and jumping have the most impact on the pelvic floor, core and joints so you want to ensure you have taken adequate time to regain strength and stability throughout the body first. It's recommended to wait a minimum of twelve weeks after delivery before running and that's only after comprehensive rehab is complete. Even if you ran during your pregnancy, start short and slow and build up gradually.

My final, and probably most important, piece of advice is to try not to compare yourself to others. Everyone has a different postnatal journey, which is affected by many factors. Please be kind to yourself and trust the process.

———

Everyone has a different postnatal journey,
which is affected by many factors.

———

Fit is fabulous

Being a good mum requires mental *and* physical strength. You need to be strong to lift up your kids, to get them in the car, to play with them on the floor . . . and you have to engage all the right muscles to be able to do it safely without hurting your back. And you need a positive outlook to get you through a testing day of begging a toddler to put their shoes on, or a tiring night with a 3am feed. Self-motivation is key . . . get started and it gets easier, but how do you get started?

I've got some old shorts that I put on every week to see how they fit. They are the shorts that I felt really good in before kids, and I remember when I first tried them on after having Wolfie, I couldn't get them over my thighs. But now I can, and it's good to keep me on track. Weighing myself weekly can also be a good way to keep me heading towards my goals. Some people join groups or sign up to apps that keep them accountable, which works well for lots of people I know. Think about what would work best for your personality. And don't beat yourself up if you can't join a gym or make it to a class: look up virtual classes on YouTube, or blast some banging tunes, set a timer and dance around your bedroom for 30 minutes. If you haven't got anyone to look after your baby, strap them to your chest in a baby carrier, or put them in the pushchair and go for a long walk. I used to walk miles with Wolfie and really work up a sweat. Half the time just getting to the gym or pulling your trainers on for a run is the hardest part. But trust me: you'll never regret moving your body. And fake it till you make it – treat yourself to some great workout gear and put it on as soon as you get out of bed, so you are ready to grab those moments to stretch or get a plank or some sit-ups in while you're boiling the kettle. I've found paying for a class or a gym membership is a great motivator too. Because you don't want to lose the money, you might as well use it. Remember, don't feel defeated if you're not an Olympian – even 10, 20 minutes a day is better than nothing. Once you start seeing the results, you'll find it easier to stay the course and complete your mission.

Food for your mood

Max is on a low carb, low sugar regime with me at the moment, which is a real help. He put on weight when I was pregnant with Wolfie as well, bless him – he didn't get the eating for two is a myth memo. He's carrying a bit of extra timber that he's determined to shift, which is good because if he was eating huge feasts and desserts, pizza and pasta, it would be hard for me to keep on track. We aren't too strict, though. We're not miserable, and still have naughty meals – I love a chicken jalfrezi and all Indian food, it's why I called my daughter India (I'm joking!) – and will have a few glasses of champagne if there's a good reason to, although obviously tequila is better for people watching their calorie intake. We're being healthy but it's obviously really important to live at the same time. So, give yourself your cheat days. I don't tend to eat carbs every day but smash loaves of bread if we're having our cheat day. You can't be sensible the whole time. But after a blowout, Max and I agree, 'Let's not do that for a while' – for my anxiety as much as my waistline. I feel so much happier when I've eaten really healthily for a week or two, and then if I fancy a few drinks and a cigarette, I'll treat myself and get it out of my system. Remember what Mummy Felstead says, 'Everything in moderation' – even the sensible dieting and exercising bit! If you have hard and fast rules, you'll feel guilty and anxious every time you break them, and life is too short for that. We're not bodybuilders! But

I've done my fair share of partying and I don't want to deal with hangovers as a parent . . . which as I've said, isn't really a traditional pukey-headache of a hangover now I'm in my thirties, but an anxiety attack. It's just not worth it. My drinks of choice these days are more likely to be large bottles of water and protein shakes.

We've got a meal preparation company delivering healthy ready-made dinners to us now, which are really easy and delicious – and a lifesaver when you've had a baby. Cooking (and cleaning up afterwards) is just another thing to think about, isn't it? It keeps us on a healthy, well-portioned track too. You're more likely to overeat if you're serving yourself, whereas if it's prepared for you, it's all measured out. If I'm hungry in the evening, I go up to my bedroom where I've hung up a favourite item of clothing outside the wardrobe that I'm desperate to get into and look at it. It stops the snacking. Or I just think about the summer holidays and imagine myself in a bikini. Just work out that happy, balanced place between starving yourself, which won't work long term, and overeating. Don't ever let yourself go hungry, but don't mindlessly eat because you're bored or depressed.

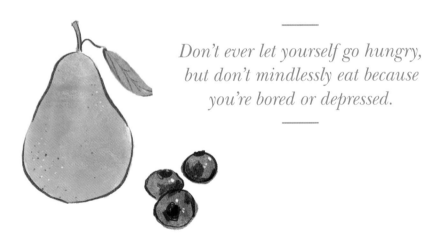

Don't ever let yourself go hungry, but don't mindlessly eat because you're bored or depressed.

THE IMPORTANCE OF
EATING WELL AS A NEW MUM

JOANNA LENZ, DIETITIAN

As a new mum it can be really hard to prioritise your own nutritional needs. Personally, I hadn't done the whole 'prepping meals and freezing them' beforehand. I was working full-time two weeks before I gave birth and was too exhausted! It's amazing if you can, but not everyone feels like batch cooking in the latter stages of pregnancy! When I had my first baby it was such a shock to the system I relied heavily on support with cooking. My mother-in-law would bring dinners, my mum would make lunches and other meals but when my husband went back to work it was even harder. Eating enough fibre is important so you don't get constipated. When you're recovering from birth this is definitely something you want to avoid. A new mum's iron levels will return to normal provided mum is eating a well-balanced diet with plenty of iron-rich foods. Lack of iron can lead to tiredness and low mood.

Even as your children get older it can be difficult to eat well and maintain a balanced diet (I know this only too well having three children). I can be found preparing wonderfully balanced home-cooked meals for the girls, fruit platters with all the colours but then find there is none left for me! It's easy to forgo a meal for biscuits, caffeine, cake at soft play and even though I'm a dietitian, this happens all too often. Don't get me wrong, I love to cook but when you're the one doing all the cooking for everyone, every day – sometimes you just don't feel like eating it. Even when I do sit down at the table to eat, invariably someone wants something, so up I get again. It's good to set boundaries and let your children know that you need to eat too. Eating together as a family is something I always advise, even when you start weaning – baby needs to learn from someone!

Food for the future

I have to be careful about talking negatively about my weight, my body image and my eating habits in front of India. I am aware that I am a role model, and she looks up to me to copy how I talk about my shape, which in turn could affect her self-confidence in the future. As a family, we make an effort to have fun in the kitchen, to have fun outdoors, to move a lot, to dance. I lead by example to show the kids how fun it is to cook at home and how delicious healthy food can be. We make smoothies with cinnamon, peanut butter, spinach or blueberries – whatever we can find. I have such strong, wonderful memories of my mother's Sunday dinners growing up, all the vegetables you can imagine smothered in her amazing gravy, and a humongous roast chicken. Then she'd boil down the bones to make a delicious stock and we'd have this warming, nourishing chicken soup the next day with any leftovers. I loved those meals, and I want to replicate that feeling for my children. I cook a roast chicken every week now, the smell filling the house, and we eat the meat, then I use the stock for a vegetable soup – and I even put the stock in Wolfie's bottles. Yes, it sounds off, but he loves it and bone broth is so good for us. An older kid would probably think it was yucky, but Wolfie is too young to push it away.

———

I loved those meals, and I want to
replicate that feeling for my children.

———

EASY WAYS TO EAT WELL

ADAM SHAW, CHEF, AUTHOR OF *HOW TO GROW YOUR FAMILY* AND FOUNDER OF AT DAD'S TABLE

It's really hard sometimes to eat well when you're also making three meals a day for the kids, supplying them with endless snacks and trying to cook the fine line between making food that meets both their nutritional needs and yours. Here's a few hacks:

1. **SWAP YOUR CARBS.** Little people need carbs for energy and to help them grow whereas carbs can make older people just feel bloated. To give them the best quality carbs and reduce bloating, swap starchy white bread and pasta for wholegrain, brown for white rice and sweet for traditional potatoes.

2. **COOK ONCE, EAT TOGETHER.** If you can, cook once for the family and eat together around the dinner table. This will stop you eating a full meal later while also polishing off the kids' leftovers, something we are all guilty of doing (who isn't partial to the odd fish finger?!). Plus, you'll save time and eating together is best for inspiring food confidence in youngsters as well as better family bonding.

3. **EATING WELL DOESN'T HAVE TO BE COMPLICATED OR EXPENSIVE.** Use up wilting bags of greens by making your own pesto (olive oil, garlic, nuts, cheese and spinach/kale/basil/rocket), add a drained can of lentils to a spaghetti/chilli/cottage pie, add a spoonful of chia seeds to porridge and add a cup of frozen peas to a boiling pot of pasta.

4. **UTILISE BATCH COOKING TO FREE UP TIME AND REDUCE SNACKING BETWEEN MEALS.** Get into the habit of making double portions and freezing the leftovers, so when you're short on time you've always got a nutritious choice in the freezer. As well as pasta dishes, casseroles and stews, stir-fries, soups, tagines, risottos and pie fillings are all great options for the freezer.

FUELLING UP

RO HUNTRISS, DIETITIAN

Motherhood can be a tiring time and when we are tired, this is often when we don't make the best food choices for our overall health and wellbeing. While a quick snack on something less healthy might seem like an easy and convenient way to get some quick energy, these choices may not be supporting us longer term. The prospect of eating well and prioritising yourself can sometimes feel daunting, especially when you are busy. It may seem that there aren't enough hours in the day. But the most important thing as a mother is to not forget about yourself.

Making time to create a nourishing diet for yourself can help you to feel more energised and support your mental health, putting you in the best position possible to face the challenges that motherhood throws at you. Opt for whole grains over refined carbohydrates, these release energy more slowly across the day, helping to support and sustain your energy levels, which is important, especially when you are juggling the many aspects of family life. Aim to plan meals for the week for the whole family, so you will know what you are going to eat every day and you will have the ingredients ready. Take nourishing snacks with you when you are out so that you don't end up grabbing a quick snack that may not be as supportive of your health and have nourishing foods, such as a filled-up fruit bowl, at home.

The most important thing as a mother is to not forget about yourself.

Memories to feed the soul

I love cooking in big batches, and it's turned into a cute little routine with India. We turn on some Madonna – preferably *The Immaculate Collection* – and chop and blend and bake. Her favourite thing to make together is banana pancakes. She will crack the eggs into the pot, and stir in all the other ingredients, then we sit down to eat them, and I tell her how delicious they are and what a good cook she is. I still remember the pride I felt when I made a cup of tea for my parents for the first time and being told how yummy it was. Yes, it was a ploy to get me to bring them tea more often, and I fell for it, but there is something really nourishing about a family that cooks, drinks and eats together – and doesn't push food into a shameful spot.

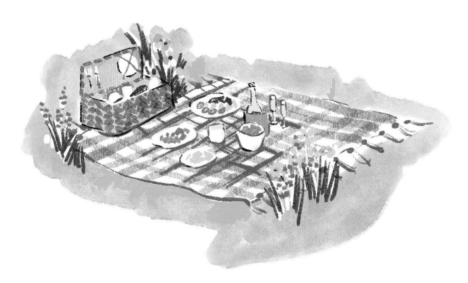

CHAPTER SEVEN

Self-care and Soul-savers

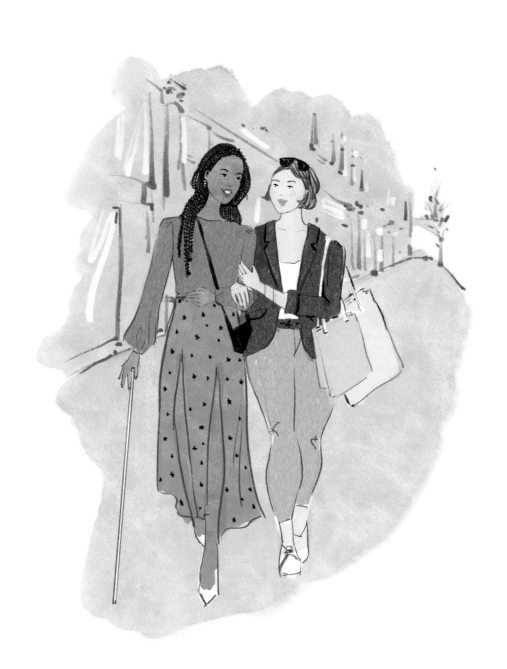

Investing in wellbeing is important for everyone, not just mothers . . . but *maybe* especially mothers, right? It's something that I didn't know about or do for myself for a long time, not properly anyway, not in a meaningful way. I grew up watching my incredibly glamorous granny Baba, my mother's mother, who would invest time and money in herself, but it was all very external. I'd visit her at her home on Richmond Green, and sit with her in her bathroom, where I swear, she had a thousand different luxurious creams, lotions and potions covering every surface. She was the Queen of Self-care – if it can be measured by how much money you spend at beauty counters – always wore huge sunglasses and lectured me that 'A woman must always take care of her face,' while I watched her slather, dab and rub, mesmerised by her indulgent morning routine.

My mother was the same, doing things to look after herself, but more for appearances than inner wellbeing. She never went to the gym; instead I used to sit and watch as she attached herself to a machine that she swore would wobble the fat off her. She'd shake away while reading the newspaper or drinking a cup of tea, strapped up to this modern, miracle contraption. She'd play a spot of tennis with her friends as well, but they'd follow it up with a few bottles of champagne afterwards. She very much had a traditional sense of what a woman needed to be in that era, focusing on her husband and children more than herself. Every evening, she'd know exactly what train my dad was catching from London's Victoria station, and rush upstairs to put make-up and nice clothes on for him, dinner in the Aga waiting. She and her friends would rush upstairs for their men and say, 'I'm going to put my face on!' Poor Max is lucky if he returns from work and I have clean hair.

These ideas of self-care being made up of external things continued when I was on *Made in Chelsea*. I used to get a spray tan once a week because I don't tan, and I took the time to get these – with hindsight – awful extensions put in my hair. Because the rest of the cast were so beautiful and fashionable the show producers pretty much told me to step up my game on the glamour front – and I did . . . until I became a mum, and I realised that too often we confuse these external treatments and vanity projects as self-care, and they are a treat, but the more long-lasting, beneficial self-care is the stuff that allows your buzzing brain to quieten, your tired body to replenish itself, your lacklustre soul to be lifted. I still consider getting my roots done and my nails varnished as a lovely luxury, but today self-care goes a bit deeper . . . and often involves a good night's sleep.

———

The more long-lasting, beneficial self-care is the stuff that allows your buzzing brain to quieten, your tired body to replenish itself, your lacklustre soul to be lifted.

———

Making yourself a priority

When you become a mum, it can come as a shock that you're no longer your number one priority. You fall down the list of what is important. But please, make time for yourself. Even 20 minutes a day can make a big difference to how you handle the other 23 hours and 40 minutes you're faced with. Even taking a few minutes before bedtime to make some notes about your thoughts and feelings in the journal section at the back of this book could help remind you to value yourself! Try it now – note down some things about your mothering experience you love or want to change.

My biggest boost to self-care is the time I spend on my fitness, which I talked about in the previous chapter. Just this morning, I didn't want to get up early to go to the gym, I felt low and had zero spark about me, mainly because Max and I are like ships that pass in the night at the moment and that pisses me off . . . but I made myself go to the gym, knowing – although I *really, really* didn't want to go – that just an hour on my own, working out and feeling strong, would boost my mood all day long. And it did. I got a sweat on, listened to some uplifting music and lost the bad mood. I know myself: I am insecure, I do have my demons and I can overthink everything, so I take every opportunity I can to get myself into a positive headspace. Believe me, you never regret going to the gym.

I project happiness and strength when I've invested in myself, which makes me a better mother and more attractive to Max, and I don't mean physically but emotionally. My default position is to be a bit needy and pathetic when I'm not in tune with myself, which is so unattractive. Honestly, I cringe when I think about some of the tragic conversations I've had with ex-boyfriends. I suppose I've always had a problem comparing myself to the cool girls around me, and I have never been cool. As a kid, I had big round glasses, train-track braces and I had the worst acne when I was in sixth form – to the point I had to keep a concealer in my bra in case I brushed past someone and the make-up came off to reveal a red streak of skin. My look before my twenties – well, my family and I called it 'God's natural contraception.' Then on the show I was never a sex symbol like some of the other girls, even though the glasses, braces and acne were long gone, and I got cheated on numerous times so still didn't have a deep grounded sense of self-worth. Still, it was around this time, watching the lives of my other castmates and their interactions with other people, that I started to understand that it didn't matter how good you looked on the outside, it was more important to feel good on the inside.

Family matters

My greatest fan, and the saving grace for my fluctuating self-esteem, has always been Mummy Felstead, my biggest cheerleader, and a good ally to have around when doubts creep in. I hope there is someone in your life who always has your back. We need solid family – or framily – to strengthen our roots in self-belief and strength. When I moved to London and got a little house with my two girlfriends from school, we had a tiny spare room and Mummy would come and stay whenever she wanted – which is unheard of, I know! What normal people want their mum to come and stay and party with them in their twenties? But she was my firmest advocate, for ever telling me how amazing I was and how proud I made her. I guess I didn't take all of it on board, because I thought that's what mums should say to their daughters,

SELF-KINDNESS

CHERYL MAY NDIONE, FOUNDER OF CONNECTED
CONSCIOUS AND CERTIFIED WELLBEING COACH

We're conditioned to believe that we're an unreliable source, and it robs us of our brilliance. If so many of us rely on external forces, be it the subtle messages from society or unsolicited advice, we can very often feel stressed, inadequate and overwhelmed by trying to get things right. As a result, our wellness takes a back seat because, let's face it, there's not really any downtime as a mum unless you feel you deserve it, create it and prioritise it.

We must take steps to tune back into what our mind and body need day to day. My work is to support that deep connection to self that often gets lost along the motherhood journey. It is actually this connection to self that has led me to listen to my physiological cues and has allowed me to move freely through the world, without guilt, living a life that feels fulfilling, self-determined, and in line with what I believe to be best for everyone.

I say all this to highlight that self-trust, self-belief and self-assuredness in your ability to make the right decisions for yourself and your family will put your life on a path that might feel rebellious, but will ultimately lead you to satisfaction and will help you to be a beacon of light to those that need it most. It's not selfish to prioritise your wellness. It's sensible. Life is short. Do your duty. Protect your family. Trust your instincts. Live your life! You're someone's child too! You deserve to be looked after!

*It's not selfish to
prioritise your wellness.*

but it was nice to hear. I know she didn't get that when she was young, and maybe because of that, she does have a deep-rooted lack of confidence, and didn't want me to experience the same. She had a very tough upbringing; her father died when she was very young, and her mother married again, and became one half of a very glamorous party couple, always at country clubs and country houses. An only child, Mummy was very lonely. She has memories of being left in the car in the grounds of country manors at night for hours and hours on end, while her mother and stepfather would go inside and be fabulous. It all left her quite insecure. And then she married my dad . . . and, as you know, that ended in a difficult divorce.

Finding myself in motherhood

After all the shenanigans of the show and celebrity, having India to care for was a breath of fresh air. I had a purpose. I had stability. I had something that was mine, that I had to grow up for and look after. She was my everything and I suddenly found I didn't care about the silly little things any more, like cheating boys, boozing, what other people thought about me. She made me care about myself more, ironically, from a wellness point of view. I wanted to be fit and healthy for her. I'd spend more time out in the fresh air, taking long walks, appreciating the changing seasons, teaching her about nature, eating well and making the effort to work out when I could. You're never going to regret a long walk blowing away your cobwebs, either. Max and I often say to each other when we feel tension in the house that we need to get out of the four walls, together or alone, to slow down and breathe again.

An attitude of gratitude

I struggle with the whole meditation thing, but I know many mums really benefit from that to start or end their day in a calmer state, so try it out – there are so many apps and online videos that can help guide you. Max and I do our own *sort of* meditation, which is to repeat daily affirmations, putting grateful vibes out into the atmosphere. It's quite spiritual. I always say thank you for everything I have at the end of the day, before I go to sleep. That's really important. Many studies have shown just the simple act of gratitude or saying thank you boosts your wellbeing so much and it's such a simple thing that we could all do. And of course, I'm aware that I am very lucky and have lots to be grateful for, but even in times when I haven't, there's always something isn't there? Someone loves you, or someone is speaking kindly about you, or your body is working, or you're able to pick the kids up from school and walk in the sunshine to the park. Look, there's always something.

Clearly, you can't be in a hippy, happy, peaceful state of gratitude all the time. Sometimes, just getting the kids to put their shoes and coats on can feel maddening. *Why are you testing me like this?* I think *Why are you being like this? I do everything for you, and you act like this!* And in those moments feeling grateful is the furthest thing from your mind. And that's normal. Don't feel guilty for shouting sometimes or for feeling angry or frustrated. You're a mum, not a pushover, not a servant, not a sentient being with no feelings or emotions. But just try to regroup by the end of the day, appreciate that you do have things to look forward to, or things that enrich your world.

Boundaries: self-protection

A huge part of self-care is being careful who you spend time with. You do get warning bells about people; you feel a vibe in your bones that someone is a little bit off. Your body is trying to teach you something: listen to it. Your gut reaction is important. I'm a good judge of character, I think, I can just look into someone's eyes and know if they're not what they say they are, or if they're a little bit cuckoo. I think the eyes are very important. As I've mentioned, I'm an empath, and sometimes we empaths give people more chances than they deserve because we feel bad for them, or we sense that there could be damage from something in their past. But some people can be energy vampires and leave you exhausted. Drained! Limit your interactions with these people. They will suck the life out of you because when someone is miserable, they spread misery. Instead, find the radiators – the people who give off warmth and draw you to them, the ones who radiate cosiness and comfort.

YOUR INNER CHILD

Once, when I was having counselling, I was put into something that felt like a trance – it was amazing, it felt as if I was about to start levitating – and the therapist started talking about how we've all still got the little boy or girl we once were inside of us, and if you can imagine them crying you can then work out how to comfort them. When you've done some of that work, the therapist said, you'll learn how to be kinder to your adult self. It would be lovely if we could climb into a big bubble and wear it as a shield of armour every time we went out into the world, letting all the negative energy just bounce off us. I try to visualise that, to stop bad stuff getting to me, looking after my inner child. You could say affirmations which would soothe your inner child and the you of today, too.

You need to talk to yourself like you would talk to a friend. Would you ever say something cruel or mean to a friend who is crying, even if they've done something really quite stupid? Never. You wouldn't. You'd be like, 'It'll get better. You'll be fine. You've got loads going for you. I love you.' You need to talk to yourself like that: how you'd talk to a child or a friend.

Reducing the angst in anxiety

My anxiety is easier to handle these days, now I've got a better routine. Now I'm a mother, getting woken up in the night and never knowing if a tantrum is around the corner. I can't go back to knocking back the cocktails and risking thousands of things whirling around in my brain, keeping me up all hours like they used to. If I do get an annoying attack of the angst, a session at the gym or a long walk does wonders – even if I don't feel like going at the time.

Max has found a really good way to plot our goals, aims, things to look forward to – individually and as a family, which really helps me know what is what, and lessen my anxiety, too – he gets us to do spider graphs, which we pin up in our office at the end of our garden, and look at every day. It helps us to be positive, think about the future, and it gets me out of my head and helps me see we're taking big steps in the right direction. I tick things off as they happen. It's really lovely seeing, at the end of the year, what you've made happen and what you've accomplished. Try it out – writing your plans down in a journal, or doing a mood board, or even something as simple as a to-do list. It gives a worrisome mind something constructive to focus on. It limits your ability to get side-tracked by drama or worry.

One thing Max could do better with is being tidy. I find great peace in having a neat, clean home. Max is mostly good, but let's shit build up on a particular chair in our bedroom and leaves his socks on the kitchen table, and I can't tell you how crazy it makes me. He lived in Hong Kong for seven years, where cleaners charge about $3 per hour, so he's used to having someone running around picking up his clothes and it's the one thing we regularly argue about because messiness makes me stressed. Max – I hope you read this and start putting your clothes in the laundry basket or putting them away!

Sleep hygiene for happiness

I can't nap during the day. Whenever I've tried, I've woken up very low, almost depressed. Even after a rough night up with the kids, I can't do what so many experts advise, which is to catch up on sleep during the day, while they're sleeping or at school. If you can, more power to you – go for it. If I need to switch off and have a lie-down, I'll watch bubblegum television or read a Jilly Cooper on the sofa. Getting off social media is really important for a proper chill out, especially before bed. Being glued to a phone makes everyone's anxiety worse. Switch it off for self-care if you can at least an hour before your bedtime. Another sleep tip is to take a bath – as a filler for sleep (I often take a long, relaxing bath in the afternoon just before I get the children), or before bed. A warm bath with essential oils is very therapeutic. We're all bath people in our house actually, and it helps all of us to take that step from a busy day to a restful night. I jump in with the kids sometimes, which is fun for us all. That's when India and I have our best conversations, when she can get anything worrisome off her chest before bedtime.

Handling the grind

Even after five years of motherhood, I'm still bad at being woken up at night. Every night, when the moon is out, I'm a complete bitch, to the point Max knows it and is more than happy to get up and help because he knows there's just no point dealing with me after a badly disrupted sleep. Luckily – even after a really bad night – I'm a really good morning person. I put it down to having to get up at 7am every day to muck out my horses as a child. But don't for a minute think that means I have my shit together. I don't. No one does. But if I'm feeling really shit and out of control, I just have faith that life is going to get better because I'm trying my best and I'm nice. Mummy Felstead always says that good things happen to good people. If you're a horrid person, you'll get bad karma. Being decent and kind helps everyone sleep more soundly. Mummy also says that everything happens for a reason, and I try to remember that I'm growing and learning from every parental dilemma or drama thrown my way.

SETTING YOURSELF
UP FOR SLEEP

CLARE YOUNG, MATERNAL AND CHILD
NUTRITIONAL THERAPY PRACTITIONER

Sleep is so important for our overall health. Our bodies heal and reset while we sleep. The amount and quality we get affects our whole body and brain. The best quality sleep can be had 90 minutes before midnight. This means you are more likely to feel refreshed the next day by going to bed earlier and waking up earlier than going to bed late and waking up late. Getting a good night's sleep for parents is easier said than done. The ideal amount of sleep is between 7 and 9 hours a night but new parents may fall short of that due to frequent night wakes, struggling to fall back to sleep and lying awake with anxiety. There are ways to give yourself the best chance of a good night's sleep.

- Try to avoid using blue light tech at least an hour before bedtime. The light will prevent melatonin levels rising, which are needed to help your brain feel sleepy.

- Keep your bedroom quiet, dark and cool. The optimum temperature is 17–19°C. Use curtains or blinds that block out light.

- Try not to do stressful or energising things within 2 hours of going to bed. This includes watching action thrillers on television or things that will raise your stress levels or exercise classes that are too energetic.

- Create a relaxing bedtime routine. You might want to take a warm Epsom salts bath (or footbath), listen to soothing music, meditate, read a book or drink a cup of caffeine-free tea. Magnesium spray is also great for relaxing tense muscles.

- Use an eye mask and earplugs, if light and noise bother you. Spacemasks are amazing self-heating eye masks that warm up for 15 minutes – perfect to help your eyes relax if you've been looking at a computer screen all day.

- Take a brain dump. If you find your mind racing with thoughts and ideas, use a journal to write down your to-do list for the next day so you don't go to bed thinking about it. Add some lavender essential oil to your pillow.

- And remember your daytime habits and activities can affect how well you sleep. Get outside during daylight hours. Spending time in sunlight helps to reset your body's sleep and wake cycles. Cut out or limit what you drink/ eat that has caffeine in it, such as coffee, tea, cola and chocolate as it keeps your cortisol levels raised (the hormone that keeps you alert) which then prevents melatonin rising to get you to sleep. Avoid drinking alcohol close to bedtime. It may make you feel sleepy initially, but alcohol can cause you to wake up more often during the night due to blood sugar highs and lows. Avoid eating large meals 2–3 hours before bed as your digestion slows down at night so you may experience bloating and pain, and it may also contribute to weight gain. Eat snacks high in the amino acid tryptophan which helps to make melatonin (the sleep hormone), oat crackers, peanut butter, a handful of nuts (almonds), sour cherries, or dairy as an evening snack.

Spending time in sunlight helps to reset your body's sleep and wake cycles.

GOOD SLEEP HYGIENE FOR
YOUR OFFSPRING

REBECCA ASHTON, BEHAVIOUR SPECIALIST,
NANNY AND SLEEP CONSULTANT

The most talked about topic among parents is sleep. How long is your baby sleeping? How early do they wake? Are they restless sleepers? Sleep is also what parents crave most. It's well acknowledged that neither parents nor children can function successfully on little or no sleep. Babies and children go through various phases of sleep as they grow and develop, and it can become a problem when a child can't settle without parental help. This is where sleep hygiene can help. The term is often used when discussing sleep practices. This involves the sleep environment and routines which are followed in preparation for sleep, both nap times and overnight. Good sleep hygiene sets the path to a better quality of sleep. Good routines create sleep cues for your baby to recognise that it's time to settle, which promotes independent sleep. For newborns, independent sleep doesn't always come naturally. Particularly at night as babies are nocturnal in the womb. Newborns also do not produce melatonin, which is also known as the sleep hormone. Melatonin starts to be produced around 3 months old and helps to regulate the circadian rhythm. Getting into a good rhythm of sleep can feel daunting at first but being prepared can really help, and it can be implemented from birth. Newborns should be getting 14–18 hours of sleep per 24-hour period, split into daytime naps and overnight sleep. Below are some good sleep hygiene practices for babies and beyond:

• Use blackout blinds to keep the room dark when sleeping and expose your baby to lots of natural light (not direct sunlight) during the day. This will aid your baby in setting their circadian rhythm.

• Read them a short story or sing them a sleepy song, and use the same soothing phrases at each sleep time.

- Consider using a white noise machine to drown out household sounds that might wake your baby. These can also mimic sounds from inside the womb, which is comforting.

- Gently stimulate your baby in short bursts throughout the day.

- Ensure your baby is feeding regularly.

- Keep the bedroom/sleep area temperature between 16 and 20°C.

- If you're using expressed breast milk when feeding before a sleep, try to use breast milk which has been expressed in the evening as this will contain higher levels of the mother's melatonin.

_____

Good routines create sleep cues for your baby to recognise that it's time to settle, which promotes independent sleep.

_____

Society and social media

Many people, especially mothers who are surrounded by noise and kerfuffle constantly, find spiritual replenishment in alone time. Not me! I like being with people all the time, but if you think you do, carve out time to be on your own – write it in your diary how you would any other social engagement. This is an appointment for self-care. My mum and Max both get their tanks filled with solitude. Mummy has always said when you start enjoying time on your own that's when you're happiest within yourself. I think that's probably true and I need to work on it. I'm always looking at ways to distract myself, getting het up about something or other if I have too much time to think or be in my own head.

If, like me, your wellness cup gets filled by being around other people, you really need to make sure they are the right people. I've got lovely, wholesome mummies and a handful of girlfriends from before I had the babies who I adore, and I've got rid of everyone else. Some people aren't true friends – whatever they declare – and realising that can feel unsettling. When you go round in life like I do, just trying to be happy for everyone, it can feel really dark when it's not reciprocated. Jealousy is a wicked emotion that crops up often, whether directed at you or your child, and you don't have time for that sinister shit. Give someone the benefit of the doubt once, but don't keep taking their sly glances or snide comments. I'm so easily rocked and unbalanced, it's quite scary. Even if I go to someone's house and it doesn't feel energetically healthy, I'll come out affected. Remember, when dealing with other people, put the feelings of your inner child ahead of anyone else's. I love meeting new people, but I don't keep them around for long if I sense something off or nasty.

Nature heals all things

As well as walking in the great, green outdoors, I think having greenery in the house makes such a difference to your mental state and sense of calm. Bringing the outdoors into your home is great for the senses – I love lighting floral, fragrant candles and having pots of bright yellow daffodils dotted around. Pots and pots of them – they make me smile when I see them. I love when spring has sprung, chasing away the chilly gloom of January and February; it's definitely my favourite time of year, although I love hot summer days with their long, sunny evenings, and autumn, too, when the scent of bonfires fills the air. I have such happy childhood memories of riding my horse through fields of wildflowers, packing picnics and exploring and feeling such a deep sense of adventure, appreciation and freedom. I felt safe and content, watching ladybirds flitting around, hearing the birds' tweets in the trees around me.

Water is another big soother for me – seeing it, hearing it, breathing it in. Going to the beach is a spiritual experience. Close your eyes and listen to the waves and you'll know what I mean. But even a pond will give you a boost! We have a wetlands centre near us which I love to take the children to; we watch geese take off in flight and make ripples in the water when they land. We're lucky to live in a leafy part of London with lovely walks, parks and the River Thames on our doorstep. Max and I have our best conversations when we go for a walk together. If he says something annoying, I can speed up or slow down a bit to take a few deep breaths while staring across the glistening water, and try not to fly off the handle, and vice versa. Being aware of the weather and its effect on your senses is a good tip, too. Feel the sun streaming through the window, listen to the rain tapping on the roof. It can soothe without taking a step outside.

Nature helps us to calm down. It's scientifically proven to do so, lowering cortisol and adrenaline and boosting serotonin. Even mucking out horse poo from stables at 7am is a stress reliever for me. Does that make me odd? Even when it's snowing, cold and dark outside, I know that is Mother Nature's way of forcing us to slow down, hibernate and light a log fire if possible!

All year round, nature really is just like the best *free* mental wellbeing tool, especially as a mother. I've found that even when children are at their most irksome and exhausting, taking them outside for exercise in the fresh air changes their mood. It helps everyone, no matter your age or ability.

I remember during the first Covid lockdown we moved into my mum's cottage in the country where I grew up, and while the world around was so sad and mad, we'd run around in the woods playing hide and seek, and when we were allowed to, we'd travel to nearby beaches and India would play with the pebbles, or we'd have barbecues in the back garden in the evenings. It was all the simplest of stuff, but India remembers it all as such happy memories, the trauma of that period in our collective lives totally passing her by. That's what good grounding looks like. Not spending loads of money on God knows what but spending time together outside. Those type of memories are the ones I look back on most fondly, and I want to create that magic for my children too. Covid has been a traumatic time for everyone, and I know lots of couples have split up with the stress of it all, but it actually allowed me the space and time to focus on what I already knew was important – family, nature and working out how you can look after yourself and the people you love in a meaningful way. I suppose that self-care has stepped into its own in the last few years. We've desperately needed to practise what made us feel good.

Hobbies, happiness and having things to look forward to . . .

We all need to escape the day-to-day grind and the miserable reality of life sometimes. Getting on a horse and going for a hack is probably the hobby that allows me to do this the most; I also love playing tennis, even though I'm not very good any more. I know lots of you love to crochet, knit, bake, draw, colour . . . whatever it is, make time for the projects and interests that replenish you. A mother can't pour tea from an empty pot! I think it's important for mothers to find something that they love outside of family and work. Women need to have something that is theirs. Hobbies can help you meet like-minded friends too, if you want to widen your social circle, and maintain your identity. Add champion potter or BMX racer to your list of attributes if it makes your heart sing and your stressed brain switch off.

WRITING YOURSELF A GREEN PRESCRIPTION

AIMEE STRONGMAN, YOGA TEACHER FOR
BIRTH AND ANTENATAL EDUCATION

Getting outside can feel like the hardest thing in the world to do as a new mum. You feel like you've travelled to the stars and have free-fallen through the portal of motherhood. Waves of responsibility hit you like tempestuous waters, and you can barely see through the fog. You ache, you are wet with milk, sweat and saltwater tears and just the thought of water hitting your body from the shower makes you recoil . . . let alone dressing yourself and the baby to brave the outside – it seems like a marathon you just don't have the energy for. Yet this is the medicine we seek; a gentle hug from Mother Nature, enveloped by the breeze to breathe life back into the new version of you.

Research has shown that the simple act of immersion in nature has a beneficial effect on the immune, cardiovascular and respiratory systems, and mood and mental wellbeing. It really is the perfect tonic for a new mama. Not only that but walking is a natural healer, massaging your shifting organs post-birth and allowing you to slowly build up strength. Being outside can also boost your oxytocin levels. This particular hormone is great for bonding with babies and for that general 'I'm feeling good' sensation. For the wilder among us, you might like to try some forest bathing post-birth or why not begin in pregnancy and build that connection to Mother Earth and all the benefits she brings. The term forest bathing translates from the Japanese practice shinrin-yoku where you take in the atmosphere of the forest and soak it all up, revelling in the benefits both physically and mentally. It has been proven to lower heart rate, blood pressure and the stress hormone cortisol as well as encourage the release of oxytocin. This has benefits not just for you but for your baby too.

Whatever activity calls to you, I hope you can find some space to move and breathe as you journey into your new role, transforming from maiden to mother. It also helps as the children get older and being outside is part of their everyday experience! Just listen to your body – only venture outside when the time is right for you. For some that might be quite soon after birth but for others it might be a few weeks. Honour the needs of your body and remember to go slow. And remember, consistency is key – whether you walk for 5 minutes or an hour, know that if you do it regularly you will notice a difference in your wellbeing and you will feel better.

Another reason I loved lockdown was that so many mothers turned their hobbies into small businesses, hustling and bustling to create a company that worked with their lifestyle, parental restrictions and personality. They got a chance to give up the boring job they'd felt stuck in to see what else they could do with their talent. Over the last few years I've been contacted by so many fabulous mummy entrepreneurs whose confidence was bolstered by their hobbies – like a woman I know who beautifully sews names into cardigans and is smashing it in business right now. Trying out different crafts and hobbies not only gives you back much-needed time to yourself, but it helps you find out what you really love, what you are really good at. And if you can turn that into a job – into actual money – well, that's brilliant. A win-win!

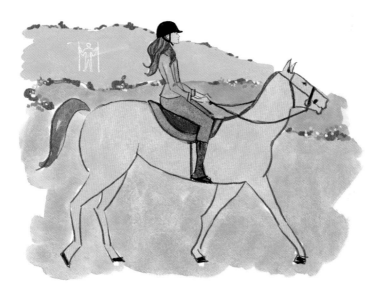

CHAPTER EIGHT

Work and Money

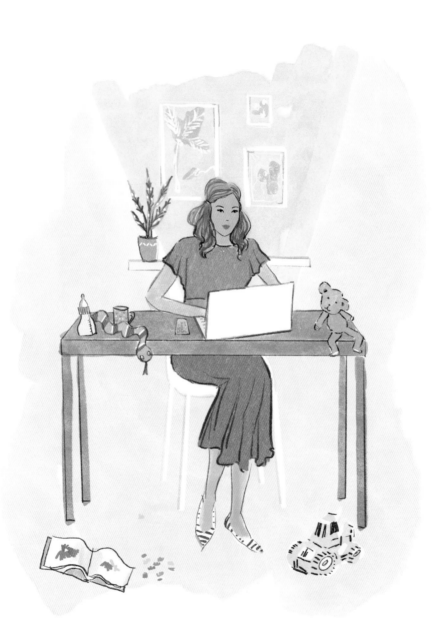

A pparently, I always wanted to be famous. My mummy and sister swear I was always talking about wanting to be a star when I grew up, and I can remember from a very young age playing scenarios in my head, imagining a glamorous, glitzy life in London for myself. Thoughts about this dream future life would send me off to sleep happy – and I think helped me manifest the life that *Made in Chelsea* gave me.

Before meeting the show producers on that night out, I had no idea what my career path would be, I had no real career aspirations, plans or passions, I was never going to be a rocket scientist or a mathematician – that was the only thing that was clear – so when the opportunity to be on camera having fun came up, I was excited. I was working front of house for a hedge fund in London at the same time, but it soon became clear I couldn't keep doing both as the show took off. I still just about answered the phone, my main responsibility, but I was always late, hungover, and sneaking off to sleep on the sofa when the bosses weren't looking. Unsurprisingly, just when the producers of the show gave me an ultimatum – make *Made in Chelsea* your all or nothing career-wise, I got fired . . . so that answered that dilemma and I leapt fully into my life as a television personality. Critics disapprove and dismiss reality television and the cast of these shows get plenty of abuse, but we won a BAFTA, and of course, the show, in a way, gave me India, because it's where I met her father.

I had no idea where it was all going, and I still don't really, not solidly, apart from Bloss, which became my first true passion project. Show business is fickle, and I'm just racing against the clock until my time fades. I'm aware of that, and don't feel sad, but it's why I started Bloss and why I'm investing in companies that I really believe in. The fame thing I wanted as a child has become less about getting dressed up for red carpets, and more about being able to lend my profile, my voice, or invest my money, to get companies that I believe in off the ground and growing. After being in the public eye for over a decade, I have amazing contacts in all different fields and worlds, and nothing makes me happier than connecting brilliant mothers to each other and helping them get a business plan together. Women certainly get a renewed creative energy once the dust settles on motherhood, I've noticed. The drive to be a good parent includes wanting to show your children what you can do, and making money to make their life comfortable, doesn't it? When India and I were on our own, she relied on me for everything, and it was empowering to make my own money, to hustle to keep a roof over our heads. And now I have Max, I'm filled with even more purpose because he is a natural entrepreneur, and I get to bounce ideas around with him, knowing he has my best interests at heart, and we are making financial decisions for the four of us as a family.

Boss after baby

The decision to go back to work – or not – after you've had a baby is always going to be a difficult one, no matter who you are and where you work. Sometimes your confidence might be dipping after months of little sleep, roaming around the house in a slouchy tracksuit with limited adult conversation. With either choice, living with regret and guilt will probably now be a permanent part of your daily life, even when finances dictate you must return to work, or a lack of support means you must stay at home. When making the choice, once you've looked at your budget and what decisions you can afford to make, think about what the right thing to do is for you – not just your child. Perhaps write a list of your needs and wants in the notes section at the back of this book. Be realistic about the costs of working and the loss of salary if you stay at home. Be realistic about the help you'll get from your partner, the grandparents and people you trust to look after your baby if you go back to work. Be realistic about what makes you happy and fulfilled – don't rose-tint your professional life or staying at home with your child. Neither is the easier route, neither is perfect, and both come with sacrifices. And most importantly, know that nothing is set in stone. You can change your mind if you think, after time, you went the wrong route.

THIS MYSTERIOUS WORK–LIFE BALANCE THING

I'm not sure about this mythical balance we're all supposed to strive for. Some days I'm all mum, and some days I'm all business. Getting your kids into nursery school is the most important thing if you want to strive for any kind of levelling of the work–life balancing scales, and I believe it's just as good for them to have time with their peers as it is for you to have time with yours – smart adults, colleagues to brainstorm with, people who share your philosophy.

You see these kids going to nursery when they're four years old who've never been away from their parents so they're screaming and kicking, and I think it's sad. Everyone needs to live a life outside of that tight parenting relationship. Socially and mentally, your child needs a break from you and vice versa. Time apart gives everyone a sense of agency and helps you reclaim those hours on your own to take meetings, or catch up on paperwork, or go into a store. You have to focus on what fundamentally is important. To me, it's picking India up from school, so I plan my work day around that. I'll always be there for the big moments, the assemblies, the concerts. I'm learning now that I'm a mum that there is no greater joy than putting things in the joint diary and on the calendar. I embrace routine now in a way I never did before, because it's these organisational tweaks that allow me to do the best I can for myself and my family.

I do enjoy the yin and yang of being a working mum though, especially with the work I do, which can often feel quite escapist, flitting between Mum life making chicken soup and doing the laundry and then being Binky, spoiled and pampered sitting in the glam chair at a photoshoot. I like it when I get a nice big job coming through and knowing that I don't have to panic about purpose because it's waiting in the wings, and that I can just chill and play with my kids for a few days or weeks. But I do know that most mums are not able to dictate or control their schedules as easily as I can, and I feel very lucky. Friends with stricter routines have had to firmly draw boundaries to safeguard their evenings and weekends, talking to their bosses or sharing more of the mental load with their partners. If you feel unbalanced, think about how your routine could evolve to allow you more space for what you and your children need – set some goals in the notes section at the back of the book, and work towards them at your own pace.

I enjoy the contrast of being a boss and a mother – I don't know if I could do either full-time! Remember, when I had India two days before my twenty-seventh birthday, I was a young mum – I'm still a young mum now! – so I wasn't ready, and am still not ready, just to be known as a mother. I want to be me as well. And that's what motherhood has done for me – it's given me a greater appreciation of both sides of my life. I feel grateful to have time with my kids, and grateful to get away from them for a bit to make money and collaborate with people. There's no balance. There's a fluctuating contrast. Aim for that. Some years, you might be at home full-time, buried in housework and childcare, but know that, if you want, you can change it up in time. You can make choices and changes that suit you and your family. Oh, and as a side note, I do realise most women don't have glam chairs to climb into at work, but I do think it's empowering to look your best, especially when you're having meetings or being out in the working world, so do get yourself clothes and make-up that make you feel nice. Not for your husband, partner, or boss – for you!

Letting go of perfection

There is no perfect parent, perfect boss or perfect colleague, so the idea that you could take on multiple roles and fulfil them perfectly simultaneously is simply ridiculous. Do your best, and don't beat yourself up. Things can go wrong but everyone does recover you know – as long as the good intent and stability and love is there. Take all the help you can without guilt. I think if there's an after-school club, put them in it to give yourself some extra time because they're not going to remember you not being around for an extra couple of hours. Make the moments count when you are together. Put your phone down. Look them in the eye. Listen and engage. That's all that matters.

Covid has changed so much for women, and families, especially. Working from home, home-schooling our children, appreciating what is truly important. It's been inspiring to watch so many people launch small businesses during these times, working out how to make work *work* for them, in different moments of their lives. That's why I'm not sure balance is something we should be aiming for, an even keel, a 50/50 split. I think we should be looking at when and what matters, and shaping an individual plan that could mean you're 99 per cent mummy during a dance recital day when your daughter is stressed, and then 99 per cent entrepreneur the next day when you're presenting an idea to investors. Know that it is all fluid, there is help, and that no one has it all sussed out.

Being authentic about that with the women around you will help everyone. Women are really smashing it and the cool women we've gathered at Bloss are an example of that; so many that you're learning from in the pages of this book, who've worked hard to build practices and businesses, and studied hard for qualifications, are now sharing their wisdom with the world. Our aim when we started Bloss was to build this safety net that mothers could fall into, a place where they knew they would be guided and helped to make the best decisions for their family – from how to conceive to how to find a good divorce lawyer – and I'm so proud of what we've built and the voices we have on the platform. It gives us all a community, too – for the experts and the parents who go online looking for help. Bloss helps everyone to know that they are not struggling alone, and that is built behind the scenes by a team of amazing women making shit happen.

THE TRUTH ABOUT
SUPERMUM SYNDROME

DR NATALYA FOX, DERMATOLOGY DOCTOR

Let's dismantle those motherhood myths. Colleagues will not hate you for going part-time. Only you are living your life; prioritise your life and your family above everything else. You can't do it all, all the time. There usually has to be some compromise along the way. And yes, bad days will happen. They do, but the sun will always rise again tomorrow. Remember your kids are only young once and need you the most (physically speaking) while they are still small. You have the rest of your life to focus on your career and take on more workload if you wish. Take on one new role or task at a time, and don't add more until you know you can handle the workload. Consider changing your work pattern or hours if possible. Flexitime and working from home might be an option for you, at least some of the time, and can seriously relieve any mum guilt. Write a daily to-do list of jobs, no matter how small they seem. It clears and calms the mind and helps you have a sense of achievement at the end of the day or week. And prioritise jobs in order of deadline to ensure you focus and complete the most pressing tasks first. This will relieve the stress and workload too.

You can't do it all, all the time.

RETURNING TO WORK

AFTER HAVING A BABY

TINA KAD, SPEECH AND LANGUAGE THERAPIST

It is easy to lose your confidence when returning to work after maternity leave. I felt the same when I went back to work in the stroke rehab unit in an NHS hospital, after having time off when I had my son. Being a mum, it's easy to lose your sparkle in your stretch marks . . . but, over time, I realised I actually hadn't stopped working. Yes, I'd had a break as a speech and language therapist (SLT), but I'd got myself a new job: motherhood. I learned so many skills as a mum, from time management and communication to problem solving, organisation and people management, all of which were transferable and an asset to my team.

After working for the NHS for ten years, I decided to work for my own private practice in Essex, Speech Therapy Interactive. This allows me flexibility and quality time with my son (my drive and my why), creativity in my profession and the ability to provide quality client-centred therapy. As my superpower is to help people communicate, I want to share my three top tips for finding this happy space between parenting and paid work:

- **Banish the working mum guilt,** you're a great role model. My son will see how his mum makes a difference in people's lives, advocating, helping her patients regain their independence and re-establishing their confidence and sense of being, improving their quality of life.

- **Build in flexibility and expect the unexpected.** Babies are bound to catch viruses and have teething-induced sleepless nights. Scenario planning may help you feel less stressed and confident. Babies are unpredictable and you cannot control everything. Be kind to yourself.

- **Get some support from the parenting tribe.** I have a teething baby, and a clingy baby equals a sleep-deprived mum/SLT. Many can empathise but only those that are in your shoes truly understand what it means.

Teamwork makes the dream work

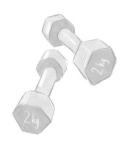

Open communication is huge at work. We have a weekly team meeting at Bloss, and then we have a follow-up call to make sure everyone knows what they are doing and can do it. And we hire good people. Make sure everyone is clear about your role in your workplace and what is expected of you. I know I'm not needed for the day-to-day stuff, but I know I'm a bit of a sounding board and mediator. Know and play to your strengths and surround yourself with people that do what you don't naturally gravitate towards. This is especially needed when you're trying to get home to your family at night – and why I think mothers are so good at this business of focusing, multitasking and knowing their shit.

It still feels weird that I'm a boss, which is probably why I joke around a lot, but that also is good as it keeps my ego in check. I never give it the big *I am*, and I don't warm to people who are like that either. All egos need to be checked at the door if you want to create something good. Own your weak spots, so your team doesn't get a bitter taste in their mouth later. When I started Bloss, I told my partner exactly what I could and couldn't do and she did the same. We laid out her map to stop confusion, too. Obviously, there are still flare-up moments and disagreements, but I have learned to remove myself from drama, take a breather, step away or put the phone down for a few minutes. I can flare up, I know myself well enough to acknowledge that, so I know when to go for a walk, have a cup of tea. I've lost friends because of my hot temper and I don't want that flaw to infiltrate my work life.

There can be a lot of emotion in business, especially for women, and even more so when you're working with friends. I know I find it hard to split everything up. I'm 100 per cent emotionally invested in Bloss and my identity is tied in with the company. I can turn on a persona of Binky Boss woman sometimes, but it feels really uncomfortable; I get this sort of back-to-school thing of feeling like people think I'm an idiot. I can get very tongue-tied when speaking in front of a large group of people and all my insecurities about not being good enough to be a boss come flooding back. And it's hard to sound articulate and together when you've been up all night with a sick kid, or you've had a few years away from the workplace while you've concentrated on child raising! I confess I have had moments working from home, trying to make sensible decisions while India is singing downstairs, and Wolfie is screaming upstairs, and I've thought *I can't sodding do this! I'm a blubbering, unintelligent mess! I don't WANT to do this!* But then, a calm would settle, I'd lower my expectations to a more realistic level, and actually use my motherhood dramas as a superpower – with all this real-world drama going on in my life, I was perfectly placed to know what mothers needed from an app!

Check in with yourself, mothers. Ask for the rules to be changed a little to help you out. Don't put imaginary pressure on yourself. And know that there's a hot bath or gin and tonic waiting for you at the end of the day.

I don't believe any mother who says everything is perfect all the time, or that she knows what she's doing 100 per cent of the time. I like the women who are open, honest, and share their struggles to help other parents – they're my type of supermums. I'm sure people have a perception of me formed through my time on *Made in Chelsea* and chat shows, from my social media accounts even, that I'm a spoiled brat who is loaded, but that's not true. I'm lucky but it's not all sunshine and rainbows. And we have to remember that about other people when doubts and insecurities about our abilities creep in. Those people who tell you – IRL or on social media – that they have their shit together and are having the best time ever might be protesting too much. Don't make their showiness weaken your ability to set goals, trust your gut or feel like doing your best isn't good enough. It is, and you are. Mothers have so much to offer to the workplace.

That's why I love the mute button on Instagram. For example, I can't handle this one woman on Instagram who has obviously got a ton of money and is always on holiday with lots of immaculate children and a doting partner, with an insane house and insane skinny girl wardrobe . . . and it's hard to see that if you're tired and feeling low. Yesterday I got called into school because India had pulled her friend's hair, and I didn't mean to, but I had a stern word with her, and then felt guilty that I hadn't handled it as well as I could have, so we hugged and cried, but it was a lot and it was exhausting and I didn't need to turn off from my at-home real life and be faced with Mrs Perfect and her angelic children. And neither do you. Block, delete, mute. Block, delete, mute. And if you ever look at me on social media and think 'God, that Binky's a smug cow,' please know that I am not, and I'm probably at that moment trying to stop Wolfie from throwing himself down the stairs and covered in chicken giblets. Curate your feeds to balance the escapist stuff with the relatable stuff, and follow people who inspire you to grow, learn, and build your business and professional aspirations, rather than rattle you with self-doubt. Mentors not mind-messers.

Empower your partner

Max does his best, but the lion's share of bath times, feedings and general running of our family zoo falls to me. It's often just easier when I do it. He does love to help, and to be home for bedtimes, cook breakfasts at weekends, but he travels more and has more work commitments outside of the home than I do. At the moment! It could all change, and the main thing is he is prepared, willing and able to step up when I need him to or when it makes sense. When your partner does help out – or, correction, does their fair share – don't over-praise (it's their family and home too!) and don't be too critical. If you are too stern and difficult, it'll put them off sharing the home workload. The world won't collapse if the dishwasher doesn't get loaded a particular way. Don't stand over their shoulder waiting to judge. When I'm tired it's nice to just take a break and leave it up to Max. And remember, it's nice for them to just be with the kids, taking charge too. They don't want to feel useless – and they're not going to learn if you don't step away and allow them to be confident in their own parenting and place in family life.

Never had it so good?

I do feel it is strangely harder for the modern woman of today than women had it even twenty-five years ago. We are supposed to be a working mother, with a tight body, flawless complexion, active social life, an even *more* active sex life . . . It's hard. But if I could give you one piece of advice it would be to focus on what is important to you, not anyone else. Choose your top two or three priorities and let the rest slide – or put them on a backburner while you work through the first few years of parenting. You don't need hobbies, or to have long *Sex and the City* style brunches every Saturday with girlfriends if you know you are happier making progress with your career and spending time at home with your kids. You do you. You can't be everywhere, doing everything. You'll end up exhausting yourself and everybody in your orbit.

I've got very good at shaving off people, places and pastimes that do not fill my emotional cup. I clear out my priorities like I clear out my wardrobe – by knowing clearly and firmly what works for me and what doesn't. Motherhood does bring stress and time constraints, but it does also bring a clarity I appreciate. If you can't wait to go back to work and have a bit of normality again, and see your old friends in the office, good for you. Find brilliant childcare and go for it. If you want a career break, go for it too. Listen to your heart – and your bank manager, HR manager and boss (information is power) – and don't feel bad about it either way, because all women are different and there isn't a right or wrong answer. Before you close off any paths, enquire about flexibility from those around you. I've had friends in situations where they have actually been really honest with their boss and worked out how to do fewer days in the office, or shorter hours so they can pick up their kids from school. There's no harm in asking, right?

And don't worry about a ticking clock. Some of my friends stayed at home until their kids were teenagers and suddenly, they got an idea, or they met someone who inspired them, and a business or second-wind career took flight. Whatever age it hits, you go for it. That's the thing: when you become a mummy you have your priorities set out properly and everything becomes a bit clearer, even though you're ridiculously tired. I keep a notepad and pen next to my bed now and just write down things that come into my head because motherhood has really given me a burst of creativity. Why not do the same? It always makes for interesting reading the next day – and there might be a genius idea in there you'd have forgotten otherwise.

BLOSS EXPERTS ON

CAREER AFTER BABY

GEMMA AND SOPHIA, FOUNDERS OF TODDLERS
TEENS AND BETWEEN, AND WELLBEING EDUCATORS

It's so good for your kids to see you work and to see how important work is to you. Whether that's in person, on the phone or on the computer, you're demonstrating what it looks like to be a working parent! We can do both and we can do it well, it just takes some planning and support. Sometimes, our kids need us in the moment, and we find the best way to ensure you're able to do both is to explain the space, place and how you work to your little one, so they have that understanding. If they want and need you for their play, start your response with a yes and say, 'Yes, mummy wants to play dinosaurs with you,' and then clarify a time boundary and say, 'Can you turn the 15-minute sand timer/click the button for 15 minutes for me to finish my important piece of work and while you wait, set up the dinosaurs? Once the timer finishes, we'll be able to play together, me and you?' Once that timer elapses, you'll give them what we like to call 'together time' and you'll pause your work and get down on their level with good eye contact and let them be the masters and experts of their play. You can use the sand timer here too!

---

*Explain the space, place and how you
work to your little one, so they have
that understanding.*

Switching gears

When I first had India, I did find it hard to concentrate on anything but her, even when I was working. Whatever I was doing – even live television – my mind would always wander back to thinking about what she was doing, eating, wearing. It was hard to be away from her, but I got on with it, and I learned that I needed my space and time to grow still. I found great babysitters who I trusted, and I got to leave the house without carrying 100 million pieces of baby paraphernalia, which was wonderfully liberating. In that first year of motherhood you can feel buried under the weight of all the new responsibilities, fears, insecurities and all the stuff you need just to care for this tiny human being for a few hours. But you must dig yourself out a bit of me time. As a single mum especially, it was important that I could just have a spontaneous dinner with a girlfriend, or go shopping last minute, and not feel too trapped one on one with India, away from adult conversation. Finding good childcare stopped me from shifting into this totally dual-focused life that I could have easily slipped into; it reminded me that freedom felt good, and who I was outside of motherhood. So much of this comes back to that old-fashioned notion of common sense again, doesn't it? Is it good for you to get away for a bit? Is it good for you to think about your own goals, aims, plans outside of your offspring? Would it be good for them to have a parent who is happy, growing and making a future for themselves as well as their family? Yes, yes and yes.

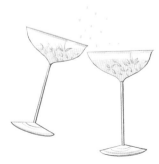

Epilogue

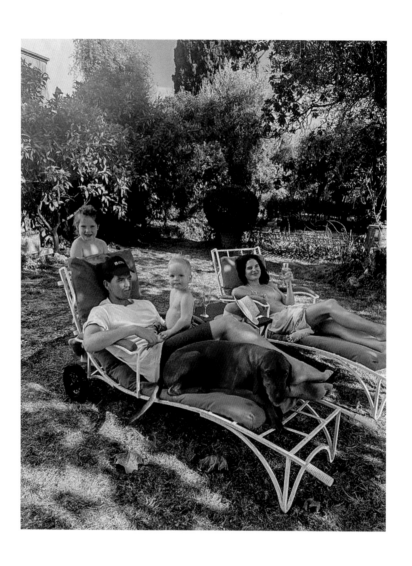

If you've thought about one thing over the hours you've spent with me reading *The Making of You*, I hope it's this: if you don't take care of yourself, you can't take care of your family . . . Value yourself! If Mummy isn't happy and healthy, it's hard for the rest of the family to be happy and healthy. And that all comes about by asking for help, forgetting perfection, ignoring judgements and protecting your wellbeing. When you become a mother, you do slip down the priority list – that's just a fact – but I want this book to be a reminder that you shouldn't fall off it completely. Be kind to yourself – and not just the *you* that is a mummy, but the *you* that you've always been. Even when you're in the weeds of new parenting, tired, unsure and stressed, it's good to remember what floats your boat, what makes you happy, what helps you to relax. Don't forget to take time out for yourself. As I've shared, for me it's working out, and not to be skinny but to be mentally and physically strong. Remember your thing and safeguard it.

And as you build your family, watch out for the things that could be grinding you down. Loneliness is a big one. Your world changes dramatically when you have a newborn. Find people who understand what you're going through, who have climbed through the other side or who are currently right there alongside you. You're not pathetic. You're not alone. Everything you've known has been turned upside down by this gorgeous, scary, cute, demanding bundle of fresh human – of course you're going to feel discombobulated. Don't suffer in silence. Talk to family, friends, your doctor, the women from your NCT classes. Read Bloss or another similar site aimed at parents. Distil your social media feed so you're just seeing helpful, honest parents sharing what really matters.

Revisiting those first months of motherhood as I wrote this book has reminded me how wonderful and overwhelming it all can be, a good reminder as Max and I start to consider having another baby, making our family bigger. I have two siblings so I've always imagined that's what my family would be made up of. I was a coil baby mistake, ten years after my sister was born, but, despite the big age gap, I love having a brother and a sister now, to get through life's dramas with. Siblings are the only people in the world who understand your parents, your childhood, the things that made you. They should be valued, and I'd love to give India and Wolfie another one.

Writing *The Making of You* has also made me realise, and I hope it helps some of you who are currently in moments of flux or unrest realise too, that nothing is set in stone. Even the worst situations can change. You truly never know what – or who – is round the corner. The difficulties you encounter as you make your family can often make you feel a deeper sense of gratitude and appreciation for the tiny victories, the glimmers of peace, and love that you share. I take nothing for granted. I remember the fears, doubts and worries I felt as a single mum, me and India against the world, not knowing if I'd ever meet someone special. And then came Max. Don't get me wrong, we can argue like cat and dog, and I can be stubborn and he can be a dick, but I know he loves me and India with everything he has. And Wolfie cemented all that. The family we have made might not look like the traditional, expected family, but we have made it work for us . . . beautifully.

I can't regret anything in my life, because every mistake, misstep, moment has got me here, to these three people. The tough times have helped me grow up and learn; I'm a better person for not wafting through life with ease. I still have times when I feel utterly shit but, on the whole, I feel very lucky and content. My past also informs the future, my expectations are realistic. I'm dreading the teen years when all those extra hormones will be clashing around the house. I was a pretty naughty teenager, so Mummy Felstead laughs that I'm going to get payback for her suffering from my own adolescent children. I'll definitely appreciate Max's cool-headed calmness when those years kick off. I trust his opinion so I will happily leave a lot of those decisions on raising teens to him. It's such a treat having a partner you respect!

And that is such a huge part of making a family that works. Respecting everyone's place, opinion, needs and wants. Being a unit. Communicating. Everyone has an equal stake in making it work. You can't pull all the weight, do all the things alone, hoping and praying for everyone else. A family is a team, each member having as much to gain from its success or lose from its failure as everyone else. I believe it's the most important team you'll ever be a part of, and it should look, feel, be constructed in whatever ways work for you, not anyone else.

I know I didn't do everything perfectly; I have two kids with two different fathers, and I never got to have those heady, honeymoon days with the love of my life because I had a toddler in tow. But we'll be empty nesters before we know it, and we can travel more then, maybe even live abroad for a bit. There are no hard and fast family rules now; you don't have to follow a path set before you. We can be middle-aged backpackers, walking the globe with our backpacks on, making memories while the kids are at university. Although, if I'm honest, I feel a little tightness in my chest imagining the days when the children don't need us as much. I need to remember that feeling when they're driving me mad, don't I?

You have to make your own happiness. I remember when I got pregnant with India, I saw a few of my friends giving interviews in the press saying, 'Oh, I would never get pregnant before I got married.' Blah, blah, blah! It was a horrible thing for me to have to read people I knew and thought cared about me talking disparagingly about me like that. I took the hurt, turned it inwards, and used it to make sure I was never so judgemental of anyone else and their family or situation. As a side note, of course many of these critics went on to get pregnant while they weren't married . . . and I would only wish them well. India's arrival was the making of me, and I hope having a baby is the making of them.

A last piece of advice: be a cheerleader. Women struggle enough with self-doubt, and it gets amplified when they become mothers. Offer advice if it's asked for, but don't interfere. Share what you've learned, the shortcuts and tips, but don't be pushy. What seems hard today will feel easier this time next week. As I talked about earlier, a good friend of mine is going through some big battles with postnatal depression at the moment, but I can see her improving, getting out more, understanding what is happening, and daring to ask for help. Dark times are hard, but with cheerleaders around, willing you on, you can get through them. Be that positive person for yourself, your family and the mothers around you.

India has been the best thing that I never knew I always wanted. Please have faith that everything is going to work out. This book is called *The Making of You* for a reason: you need to put effort in. You need to build, construct, assemble, create and model the family you want. That's not easy. But nothing worth having ever is, right? Get out of your tracksuit bottoms, get out of your house, get out into nature. Put some candles on, put some chicken soup on the stove, put some music on loud and dance. Make your own luck, make your dreams come true . . . and make a family that suits you.

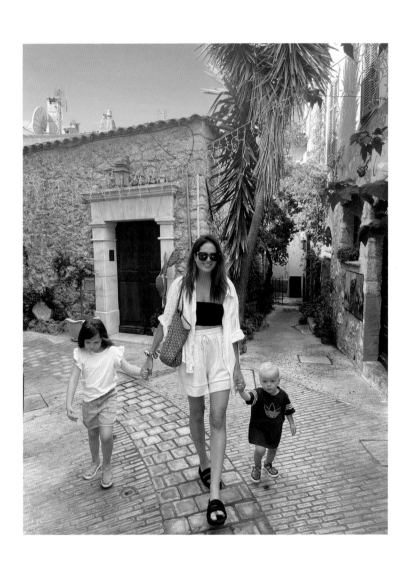

Further Resources

Check out articles, interviews and guides and find contact details for all the experts included throughout this book at **Blossapp.com**

Find more help at the following websites:

Anxiety UK: anxietyuk.org.uk

Association for Post Natal Illness: apni.org

Gingerbread, single parents, equal families: gingerbread.org.uk

Mental Health UK: mentalhealth-uk.org

Mind: mind.org.uk

Miscarriage Association: miscarriageassociation.org.uk

NHS England: england.nhs.uk

Pre and Postnatal Depression Advice and Support (PANDAS): pandasfoundation.org.uk

Royal College of Paediatrics and Child Health: rcpch.ac.uk

Saying Goodbye – support for miscarriage and baby and infant loss: sayinggoodbye.org

Stem4 – supporting teenage mental health: stem4.org.uk

Sands – Stillbirth and neonatal death charity: sands.org.uk

The National Center for Complementary and Integrative Health: nccih.nih.gov

The National Institute of Mental Health: nimh.nih.gov

Tommy's Together, for every baby – charity for babies: tommys.org

Acknowledgements

A huge thank-you to Sarah Ivens, who helped put my story so perfectly into words. You really were a sounding board and my therapist when things got emotional throughout and I will regard you as a friend for ever. Looking forward to you moving back to this side of the pond.

Thank you to the whole team at Piatkus – it has been a pleasure working with you. Thank you for turning my dream into reality. And to my wonderful editor, Jillian Young – thank you for believing in me and *The Making of You*. To my illustrator, Niki – you are incredibly talented and really did bring my visions to life in the most beautiful way.

Thank you to my Bloss team and experts. I'm so lucky to have you on board, it's such an amazing platform to help parents and parents to be, I know we are going to help a lot of people.

To my manager, Max – thank you for putting up with me and always believing in me the way I believe in you. I don't know anyone harder working and let's keep smashing it (BUNCE, BUNCE, BUNCE). And to Buffy, who puts up with a lot from me daily, who is my human tripod, children's toy builder and occasional child minder – my children now think you are Father Christmas as you always have things to bring them. Love ya, we will get that champagne on ice . . . trip to Maggie's soon!

Thank you to my in-laws and Max's family for accepting India and me and welcoming us into the family so beautifully.

Thank you to my wonderful mother for always being such a huge support. I love you.

Max, you've always believed in me and I know you are my biggest support. You always push me to follow my dreams and give me ideas. You truly are the most incredible father and role model to our children and I couldn't be luckier to call you my husband.

To my gorgeous babies, India, Wolfie and Bump (who is growing nicely in my tummy and is still a secret as I write this), you've made me who I am and you inspire and motivate me every day to be the best mummy in the world. I cannot wait to watch you grow and for our family to create lots more beautiful memories. I pray we can always talk to each other, be honest and open with each other and always stay with this close tight-knit bond that is so special. Please always look out for each other and stay the best of friends. Love you more than anything always and for ever. (I love you more than you love me.)

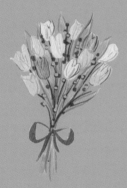

NOTES

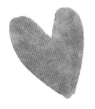

NOTES

NOTES

NOTES

NOTES

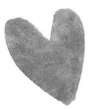 NOTES

NOTES

NOTES

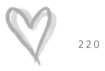

NOTES

NOTES

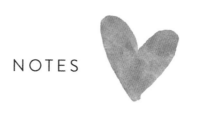

NOTES

NOTES

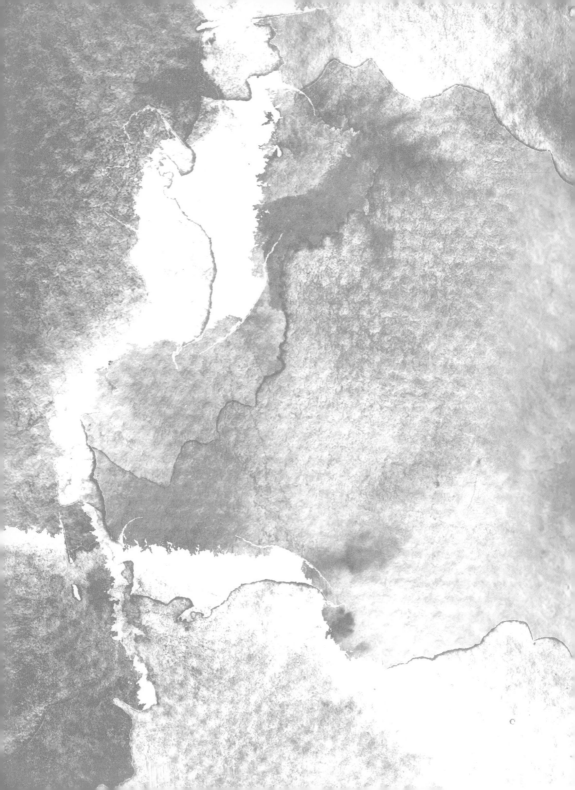